HONEY ENGLISH

A True Adventure

B. Benson

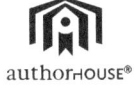
authorHOUSE®

AuthorHouse™
1663 Liberty Drive
Bloomington, IN 47403
www.authorhouse.com
Phone: 1-800-839-8640

©*2011.B. Benson .All rights reserved*

No part of this book may be reproduced, stored in a retrieval system, or transmitted by any means without the written permission of the author.

First published by AuthorHouse 12/12/2011

ISBN: 978-1-4567-6949-9 (sc)
ISBN: 978-1-4567-6947-5 (hc)
ISBN: 978-1-4567-6946-8 (e)

Library of Congress Control Number: 2011908070

This book is printed on acid-free paper.

Because of the dynamic nature of the Internet, any web addresses or links contained in this book may have changed since publication and may no longer be valid. The views expressed in this work are solely those of the author and do not necessarily reflect the views of the publisher, and the publisher hereby disclaims any responsibility for them.

Cover Photo of
Chateau de Chaban
by B. Benson

All photographs are property of the Author

Dedication

Dedicated to my Precious Daughter Genevieve, whose journey in life has barely begun… may God grant that it be filled with light and laughter, as you are my Light

ACKNOWLEDGEMENTS

Many thanks to Jim Unger, creator of the ever-endearing Herman cartoons and my next door neighbor in Nassau, for reviewing a sample of my writing and reminding me that life is not a textbook essay… encouraging me to "Dive in and make the pages come alive."

To Daniella for her utterly adamant, unbridled conviction that readers would be enticed to laugh out loud, to cry, to wonder… as she did.

To my wonderful sisters, the Catholic and the Buddhist, who enthusiastically gave these pages their blessing.

To Hanne in Lyford Cay, for the use of her splendid, and very long dining room table… when my computer failed to 'cut and paste', preferring to chew and spit. When the only way to solve the puzzle of the last chapters was to spread them out the length of the table, *see* them, rearrange them, until the optimum order revealed itself .

To Jenny, for her love and powerful prayers.

And to my daughter Genevieve…without you, there is no me.

CONTENTS

Acknowledgements vii
Of Truffles and Tempers 1
The Mad English Scientist 5
Rose Gardens and Bomb Shelters 18
From New Mexico to Monte Carlo 27
Grunion Hunts and Malibu Forest Fires 40
Of Castles and Cro Magnons 51
Banished and Beleaguered 62
Munchkins & Sky Swings 73
A Breast worth 250 Francs 87
Sailing Ships and Greek Isles 96
Greek Gods and Tibetan Prayer Flags 114
The Watusi 129
Pearls and Lace Undies 143
Drug boats and the DEA 161
The Saudi Prince 173
Of Kidnappers and Limes 181
'Windsong' and Secret Islands 192
Moi, in the Beverly Hills jail 210
Of Monks and Mystics 222
The Lord's Prayer 240
South Africa 247
The Hopetown Lighthouse 255
Forgiveness 264
Epilogue 273
Photo Gallery 279

OF TRUFFLES AND TEMPERS

This was to be, and may still be, a story of California and France, of life in a sixteenth century Castle, of nostalgic meanders among the smells of ferns and chestnut trees in the French countryside, a lifetime away from the roar of winter surf in California, the sharp tang of the sea, and the sunfilled beaches of summertime Malibu and my misspent youth. This was to be the story of how our vast tribe of seven children grew up on the beaches of one country, then traveled in glorious chaos to the gourmet heart of another, a land famous for its truffles, Foie Gras and spicy Pâté… the Dordogne.

I wanted to commit to paper the saga of the cruise ship, planes, horse trailers, buses and taxis deployed to lift us from our ten bedroom home in Malibu, along with three dogs and two horses, plus a neighboring friend of father's who didn't want to miss the move of a lifetime…all of us transported to a forty room Castle high on a hill in the very heart of France, a fairytale chateau surrounded by a thousand acres of shy wildlife, grape-laden vineyards, and seven beautiful stone houses… "One for each child," my father promised us.

It seemed future generations might like to hear what possessed Father to later donate a major portion of this paradise to exiled Tibetan Lamas, those 'venerated spiritual masters, teachers, or heads of Monasteries,' and quite different from Monks, who simply live in Monasteries.

Just give it all away…long before Hollywood turned the Dalai Lama into a household name. To the enigmatic end that we are forever linked with the propagation of Tibetan Buddhism in the heart of the French countryside. But what of his promise to his seven children to give each of us one of the beautiful stone houses on the property? That is a tale for another chapter.

For years the need to put these thoughts to paper tickled my brain, restless words tapping on the inside of my skull for a decade, begging to be let out, to feel the air, to test their strength. *Today, suddenly, the catalyst. A vicious argument, a slamming door, the angry departure of my only child, Genevieve.* My fifteen year old baby, who with her sun streaked mane of hair, long legs, wicked dimples and precocious vocabulary, passes too easily for eighteen… this juxtaposition as perplexing for her as it is for me.

She has landed herself in the heart of this true adventure, ludicrous to think any story of mine could exist without hers, as she and I are twine of the same rope.

I have shouted at her for the last time. Somehow God will have to help me keep that vow, as my temper has a life of its own; an intangible energy specializing in surprise attacks, springing from a hidden well to lash out with verbal force more lethal than any physical… leaving welts visible only to the heart. My very own temper passed on to my sweet girl, hurtling back to strike me with the force of a punch to the stomach.

The harsh words still hover in the air of the slammed door. Dazed, I seek refuge on the porch of our cottage grazing the edge of the water on this exquisite tiny island, a true gem of the Bahamas. Lost in thought, my eyes do not focus on the beauty surrounding me, I am blind. Unexpectedly I am gifted with an epiphany.

Phrases from a book I read recently flit across my consciousness. "Paula" by the Chilean author, Isabel Allende, is an impossibly beautiful story Allende wrote while her daughter lay in a coma for months, dying. By sheer writing skill, the author keeps you with her throughout the lengthy bedside vigil, intricately weaving words of warmth, love and somehow, humor.

I am reminded vividly that life may be taken from us at any moment, without warning, and suddenly I can not see the relationship with my Genevieve in the same light as a minute before; we must not part with such anger between us again.

Enlightened, my brain functioning again, the surrounding landscape bursts back into focus. The setting Bahamian sun is a smoldering globe shooting pink and orange disco lights up from the darkened sea to a graylocked sky. I turn and step back inside the cottage. Without conscious thought, I walk over to the computer, my body sits down, my fingers begin to type. Writing will fill the void until my daughter returns, will take my mind off this impasse. If only the protagonist would grace me with her presence so we can begin our New Relationship.

But what if she has decided to run away as I once did over some long forgotten teenage trifle? *Rode* away actually, on my horse in the middle of the night, tears of rage blinding me as I saddled up the mare, leaving my parents and the police to hunt half the night all over the Malibu hills, the same hills that my horse and I covered so happily in the light of day… now a scary dark place, even with a horse for company. How could I have been so brave, or such a fool.

I am amazed even now, some thirty years later, that a Malibu Police officer was concerned enough, dedicated enough, tenacious enough, to find a small girl and her horse hiding at the bottom of a deep canyon at three in the morning. Without the aid of helicopters or night lights, just one man slogging around in the dark, pushed on perhaps by the thought of his own children tucked snugly in bed. Whoever you are, wherever you are, thank you.

THE MAD ENGLISH SCIENTIST

My parents are British. Father could best be described as the perfect "Mad English Scientist", complete with piercing blue eyes hiding a surprising twinkle, and the prerequisite unruly, bushy, gray-streaked hair flying in all directions.

Father's many accomplishments were little appreciated by me as I grew up, much concerned as I was with me, myself and I. If we are lucky when we first slide into the world, we are the center of our parent's universe. When that daily shower of attention is diverted to the next sibling to come along, we are often the last to grasp that our previously 'cute' behavior has now become less than cute…if not downright annoying in the eyes of tired parents. It is somewhere in here that we embark on a lifetime of doing whatever it takes to wrest back that attention.

I digress… my first life memories begin in my father's bomber jacket, in a clawfoot bathtub devoid of water that served as a crib, in a nursery rampant with fuzzy wildlife, in a house on wheels that moved wherever my young parent's whimsy took them. Our first home as a family in England was a converted bus, the original Motor Home.

As I was not yet two years old, these earliest recollections of my own persona may not even be my own. They are perhaps but bits of stories absorbed from chats between my parents when I was older… but no, these memories are too vivid; I can *feel* the soft inside fleece of that bomber jacket as Mum and Dad wrapped me in my cocoon and gently put me to bed in the bathtub. I can *see* the texture of that certain softer, darker spot on the outside of the leather jacket where I rubbed my fingers as I fell asleep every night. I *know* the comfort of the surrounding walls of that mobile nursery, lovingly decorated with animated scenes cut from a huge 'fuzzy' book of Bambi, pasted to the wall in lifelike depictions of forest rambles.

A host of Disney characters watched over me as I lay sleeping. Happy gray Thumper and his little friend Flower the Skunk, peeking out from peaceful trees and flowers dappled by sunlight, curious butterflies alighting on curious noses… and Bambi himself gamboling on the walls throughout the various stages of his life, from a very little guy sliding awkwardly on the ice, to the magnificent stag he was to become.

My thoughtful parents omitted the traumatic forest fire scene, thereby hoping to spare me future neuroses. Yet in one of fate's great twists, we were all to relive the storybook terror in just a few years to come.

I knew father was unique, even rather eccentric in fact, but until Mother recently unearthed some old Newsweek articles praising his ingenuity, intelligence and vision, I had no idea that the messages transmitted to earth from the first U.S. space satellites were deciphered on data-processing equipment designed and built by his Santa Monica company, Benson-Lehner.

Father was a genius in a magic, fun way. Ideas simmered and glimmered at the summit of his volcanic brain, to be unleashed in steamy, showy eruptions. When California, the land of opportunity and bright sunshine called out to him, there was no hesitation. When

Britain released their emotionally shattered young Royal Air Force pilots from the hells of World War II, we were on our way to a new land and a new life.

Barely had we touched down in Los Angeles it seemed, before father dived right into his innovative world of electronics, leaving mother to wrestle with sorting out life on our explosively different planet. With unlimited enthusiasm, he deftly began designing software, hardware, data processors, computers that few people could comprehend, let alone imagine running their future world. His machines were the size of cars. He called them Ferraris, saying,

"They are so temperamental each one needs its own mechanic."

To showcase these unique creations, he bought an out of service Greyhound bus, a massive thing that had traveled the U.S from end to end with its lean greyhound logo racing alongside. Father had the bus stripped and rebuilt to accommodate his computers, and got a huge kick out of driving the remodeled vehicle around the country to technical conventions and shows. When not in use for business, the computers would come out of the bus and sofa beds would go in… and now we had a family touring bus. For trips up the coast to Hearst Castle, Santa Barbara and points North. To Monterrey and even Yosemite National Park, where a curious deer awoke us one night, kicking around the large frying pan used to cook dinner on the fire. In the morning we found the pan with its wooden handle chewed away, probably very tasty with salt from chef Mom's sweating hands.

Father had no doubt built one of the first bus/motor homes in England for his little family to live in, and now we toured the California coast in the ancestor of today's luxury rockstar buses.

How he divined such an understanding of the future, and where he developed the uncanny knack for finding solutions to problems of any size or complexity, is still a mystery to me.

The key may have been stunningly simple; to Father, 'problems' did not exist. He only saw Challenges… puzzles to be vigorously investigated and explored from all angles and perspectives. Whether solving major business questions or simple kidlet size dilemmas, he would find an answer so blinding in its clarity as to leave you wondering… "Where did that come from?"

A firefly landing in your palm could not surprise you more.

He was blessed with vision so direct and piercing that a simple question might trigger a waterfall of astounding wisdom… the twist of the cadence was so original, the final point delivered with such deft wit, it set your mind racing.

For this gift I love and admire him. And forgive the rest.

The very first story I remember hearing about Father was our little family's timely escape from war ravaged England. Age nineteen, and one of the R.A.F.'s youngest fighter pilots, Father found himself still intact as the war wound down. Stunned by the devastation being wrought, and his unavoidable participation, Father booked passage on the *RMS Aquitania* to America three years hence, for himself, a wife, and two children. When asked the names of the other passengers, Father replied, *"I haven't met them yet."*

Three years later Father and his bride sailed away from England on the pre-booked tickets, with my baby brother Christopher, and my also tiny self. Extra passengers were an English Nanny and a Springer Spaniel named *Tu Tu*. The odd name was never explained, however it was said this loyal dog one day dragged my little brother to safety on a California beach, when an oversize wave scooped him up in a moment of inattention on the part of the aforementioned Nanny. Tragedy was averted that day, only to knock harder very soon thereafter.

The trip on the *Aquitania* was only one of the great upheavals in my life, but the first and therefore scary. For the few of you who may be ocean liner history fans, *Aquitania* was considered one of the most attractive ships of her time. Nicknamed "Ship Beautiful", her opulant décor was created by the firm Mewes and Davis, who oversaw the construction and decoration of the Ritz Hotels in Paris and London. Built by John Brown and Company in Scotland, at 45,000 tons, 900 feet long and 97 feet wide, *RMS Aquitania* was the third in Cunard's Express ocean liners…she clipped along at a speed of 23 knots.

The last surviving four funnelled ocean liner, *Aquitania* survived military duty in both world wars and was returned to passenger service after each war. With 36 years of service, *Aquitania*'s record for the longest service career of any 20th century express liner stood until 2004, when the Queen Elizabeth 2 became the longest-serving liner, with an ultimate career service of 40 years.

Beautiful she may have been… but the cozy bathbed was suddenly gone, my Bambi playmates vanished, the housebus sold, our little family bundled up… and tossed upon the thunderous sea at the whims and mercies of weather and waves. Protected only by the tall, glistening steel walls of one of Cunard's finest, it was a cold, rough ride to The Promised Land.

Only a toddler, I have shadowy visions of nannies in dark coats, steamy breaths, narrow double bunks, a black and white dog, and damp, piercing cold. From subconscious memories of this grim transatlantic crossing was probably born my lifelong determination never to spend much time in places not bathed in splendid sunlight.

After leaving the cold of England, forever it turns out, except for a one year lapse when I was sent as a teenager to a boarding school in Sussex to "become civilized" (to no lasting effect that I ever noticed), we spent years frolicking on California beaches, moving to different residences up and down the Malibu coast.

On Broadbeach Road, near Trancas, we lived in a house shaped like a boat, next door to a sister creation built to resemble a lighthouse. I noticed on a recent trip to Malibu that these distinctive buildings are no longer standing; the lost landmarks fittingly enshrined in a beautiful old photograph on the wall of a trendy restaurant in Paradise Cove.

The next stop was a house on Pacific Coast Highway near Las Flores Restaurant, not far from Topanga Canyon. It was suspended out over the beach on thick, twenty foot tall pilings, the froth of hightide waves tickling at their base. One night when the rain was pelting down so hard cars were pulling over to the side of the road, a truck-sized boulder loosened by days of torrential rains crashed into our next-door neighbor's house. This muddy two story monster rock rolled down the mountainside and bounced across Pacific Coast Highway through six lanes of traffic, smashing into the neighbor's living room where it stuck, unwelcome, for weeks. Local engineers were unable to figure out how to remove the tons of rock without destroying what was left of the house, and condemned it. Our neighbors moved to a less volatile part of the country and the boulder, along with the remains of the house, were carried away bit by bit by a demolition company.

Those infamous landslides were a boon for children living up and down the coast as getting to school was too dangerous when the muddy menaces were in full force. Long stretches of the Pacific Coast Highway would be under four feet of mud for days, with huge chunks of earth breaking off forever from the steep cliff lining one side of the highway… sliding, bouncing, rolling across lanes in both directions.

Newspapers reported two white haired elderly ladies sitting on a park bench in Santa Monica at the top of those cliffs, bathed in the bright sunlight that sometimes follows a serious downpour. Chatting serenely, most likely commenting on the lovely change in the weather and enjoying their view of the ocean and deserted beach far below… they suddenly felt a strong jolt as their peaceful world fell apart. A large piece of the cliff, complete with park bench and its contents, began to slide in a deliberate and relatively smooth descent towards the tons of muck already covering the highway 100 feet below. Stunned cleanup crews wrestling with the remnants of Mother Nature's previous antics, looked up and watched the downward descent of the bench and it's passengers in horror. The bench picked up speed, began bucking and twisting, kicking up an avalanche of boulders rolling down onto those below. Time was frozen, the movie was in slow motion and God was riding with those two little ladies that day. The rollercoaster ride of a lifetime came to a slurpy halt at the base of the cliff, the bench executing a miraculously safe landing.

Cheering workers plucked those two lucky ladies from their precarious perch, their mud splattered faces registering identical amounts of shock and surprise at being in one piece.

Perhaps those very same tons of muck those lucky ladies rode down the Cliffside that day had something to do with my parent's decision to move to a safer location. They found a lovely two story house on The Old Malibu Road, facing the soft gentle bay of the Malibu Colony beach. A mile of golden sand shaped in a lazy smile, the houses and beach curved in at each end to embrace the cozy bay. At the southern end of the beach was the Malibu Pier, quite derelict, gray and rather lonely in those days. To the North was an outcrop of house-size rocks, where large, rolling swells called to surfers more courageous than I.

Behind our new house and across the lazy, 'residents only' one lane road, was a small supermarket, quite alone in a large parking lot. The very parking lot where I learned to drive. My first forays behind the wheel were on Sundays, with a brave and patient parent at my side, the supermarket closed, the parking lot deserted.

Age twelve and barely tipping the top of the steering wheel, (a thick telephone book on my seat remedied that problem the first year), round and around we went, lurching, screeching, snaking this way and that as I figured out the wiles of brakes, steering, gas pedal, and how to work them together smoothly…thanking God for automatic transmissions.

It wasn't till I lived in Europe a few years later that I tackled my first five-speed stick shift. I was thankful then to have the basics of driving already mastered, allowing me to focus solely on shifting smoothly, silently. This was the desired technique, and one to be acquired quickly with little room for mistakes, learning as I did under the watchful eye of Roberto, my Italian fiancé, in his beautiful Alfa Romeo…where grinding the gears was not an option.

Parallel parking may be an anathema to some, yet in that parking lot behind Hughes Supermarket, I became an ace. Perhaps it was father's love of the 'angle of the fandangle' that passed on to me, or perhaps I just had a knack for it. The high score on my sixteen year old driver's test was due to the examiner being suitably impressed as I slid backwards smoothly, perfectly, into the small marked space.

The old Hughes Market, with all its childhood memories for me, is still there. The landmark is now enveloped by the sprawling Malibu Shopping Plaza, a place I love to visit. Designed with care and flair as an upscale shopping and lunching refuge for residents and visitors alike, it is spiced with casual outdoor Cafes, shade trees, flowering bushes, and comfy benches. Swings for the smaller children garnish the happy plan. Unharried parents, some famous some not, lunch in relative peace, with eyes on the kidlets, mouths on the food.

One last Malibu move. We are getting numerous now, seven towheads and assorted animals. The simple word 'move' is becoming less appropriate. Something fraught with angst and chaos would be more seemingly. To tell the truth I have no memories of 'moving stress', only the excitement of each new house. This is one of the high mysteries of childhood. My exceedingly capable mother would be the one with whom to talk of moving angst and chaos.

Off we trekked one last time, bag and baggage… Bedouins with gas-fueled camels, a few doors up the road to The Big House, as we kids called it. Here under the rose garden, the bomb shelter would be born.

The house encompased two floors of large airy rooms woven into one grandiose home by a wide, curving staircase. The playroom downstairs boasted a full size pool table, built-in saltwater aquariums, and walls of mirrored shelves; shelves my sister Jenny and I claimed as our own to display numerous trophies and ribbons won at local horse shows. My little brother is no longer with us, but I cannot speak of that yet.

The enormous kitchen was the busiest room in the house. Mother presided over this aromatic airspace with calm and inventiveness. She was assisted by Rosa, our ever smiling, ever patient Spanish housekeeper. Rosa came to live with us after the nanny returned to the cold mists of her English childhood.

Mother whipped up tasty meals with alacrity for dozens of hungry faces, numerous times a day, feeding not only our large brood, but often loads of our friends, cohorts ranging in ages from tots to teens.

To my memory she also handled with much charm and no rancor the business associates Father brought home to dinner with little or no warning, cheerfully scaring up delicious meals from an apparently bereft larder. On the subject of the tasty meals Father would assuredly agree, on the lack of consequences, he might not.

This was a house of laughter, a house of pranks. One night father's glass of red wine was secretly replaced by an identical one with red food coloring and water. We watched in glee as his eyes widened with amazement, and yes… fear, as he began shouting, *"I've lost my sense of taste, I can't taste anything!"* What hilarious sport to watch him writhe on the floor, beating the carpet with his fists in the agony of thinking the luxury of taste was gone… ever the Drama King.

We kids had not expected such a heartfelt reaction however, and very soon just couldn't take it any longer, avowing the filthy deed. Watching his anger at being tricked so beautifully turn to relief that his taste buds were intact, then the uproarious laughter… that was something to remember.

Father was often asked if he was Catholic, given the large number of children. He would chuckle appreciatively and respond with a wicked grin, "No, I'm Passionate Protestant!"

Before my parents divorced, before father married my Paris roommate Maritee, had three lovely daughters and brought the total to ten… there was the original brood of seven. A new blond little cherub was born roughly every other year until we reached three boys and four girls, at which point my mother said to my father, 'Enough, if you want more, have the next one yourself."

Actually she had eight children, if you count our beautiful little Christopher, allowed to stay on this earth only until his second birthday, when life was wrenched from him by negligent nurses and doctors in a Santa Monica hospital.

Being a parent now myself, I don't know how any parent lives through such a loss. I'm sure it affected my young life, and that of my unborn little sister Jenny, waiting in my mother's womb of misery and grief, to be born with the daunting task of replacing that which is irreplaceable.

Years later Jenny sought those answers, finally putting to rest much that had been puzzling her about herself. Only two years ago, she was able to talk about Christopher's death with our mother for the first time, something I can still not do to this day.

Mother said Christopher had gotten a small pebble lodged in his nasal cavity, and was put under general anesthetic to remove it. Hours later, Christopher had not woken up and my mother was frantic.

In her early twenties and newly arrived from England, her pleas for assistance were tempered with politeness to the doctors and nurses whom she had been taught to respect, although her instincts were screaming, "Something is wrong, something is dreadfully wrong!"

She could see Christopher was not breathing properly. For six hours she rocked him, hugged him and sang to him. The nurses stopped by only long enough to say, "He will be fine dear, he will wake up soon."

Christopher never did wake up, he turned blue and died in my mother's arms. In the ensuing confusion and panic by the hospital to cover up the terrifying negligence, (or was it murder?) of a sweet, innocent and perfectly healthy child, the little body disappeared. There was no funeral that I remember, and no outlet for the grief stricken parents or myself, his little sibling.

My sweet Goldilocks girl has not come home. Although listening intently for every whisper or imagined footfall, I am nowhere near the point of handwringing worry for her safety; only anxious to set things straight.

I have chosen this corner of the world in which we now live because it is truly a haven. The days are blessed with golden sunshine and emerald waters, the nights so clear the galaxies are bright to the naked eye. There is safety in the sharp light of the moon, spinning its cycle from the thinnest slice to a full pie, often looming so close that ever-changing scenarios are definitely visible on its imperturbable face.

The year round residents here are gentle people, politely uptight as only the British and their descendants can be. Visitors are so pleased to find this little bit of heaven that they leave any bad habits or meanness at home, and become one with us… walking the tiny pedestrian paths, happily greeting all with a smile and a hello.

There is no crime here; doors are left unlocked at night, bicycles sit unconcerned on sunset-oriented porches, awaiting tomorrow's adventures.

Blossoming potted plants sway outside the local grocery all night, sweetly perfecting enticement skills for daytime shoppers; greenhouse puppies eager for a home. This is a miraculously safe place to live.

So it is not Genevieve's safety I am worried about, only the unresolved bitterness between us. And this is my punishment, being made to wait, impatient and full of good resolve while she takes her own sweet time to cool down.

Write. I will write and write, an anchor to keep me calm. I will not dash off looking for her yet, typically self-centered, ready to make peace whether it suits her or not. Changes will be better wrought by weaving our two colorful personalities together to make one harmonious fabric. I can do this, I can wait.

ROSE GARDENS AND BOMB SHELTERS

My mother loved to ride horseback. Somehow she found a way to put the trauma of losing a child into a quiet place within herself, a place that did not disturb outwardly her enjoyment of the new ones that came along in rapid succession. She was happy to share her enthusiasm for riding with us, and had been tossing my sister and I up on horses on various ranches in the Malibu area when we were still too little to let the horse know who was boss, which resulted in several near catastrophes.

Before we had our own horses, we rode every weekend at a little ranch perched on a hilltop in Latigo Canyon. My little sister Wendy was about three at the time, riding a nice old gray horse one day at a lazy walk around the elliptical ring, when the mare suddenly awakened from a horsy daydream to find she had almost no-one on her back.

Perhaps she had a malefic glimpse of her ultimate demise, or simply thought in her horsy old way, "Life is passing me by!! It's now or never, I'm making a bid for Freedom!" Whatever the obfuscation, with a spurt of heretofore unseen energy, the Old Gray Mare clambered purposefully over the wooden fence surrounding the little riding ring cut into the side of a mountain. Making short work of the rickety posts and rails, the mare snorted a breathy whinny, and began mountaineering up the side of the steep hill. My tiny sister was holding on grimly for dear life, appropriately puzzled that her usually flat world should now be tilted straight up above her.

Mother and I froze in a learned reflex guaranteed not to startle a horse...startle her? She had wings! In this 'calming mode' we mouthed soothingly to the fleeing horse, "Easy there, whoa now, take it easy girl." Useless placations that rose to the lips before consultation with the brain. Heading for the summit, more preoccupied and determined than at any other time in her life, the mare ignored us completely.

The owner of the little ranch was a Hopi Indian, a gnarled old nut of a man. Luckily he was not repressed by the conventional methods he had taught us. Reading no doubt more accurately the larceny glinting in the flashing eyeballs, he sprinted quick as a deer up a dirt path to head off the duo, snatching my sister to safety just as the mare made her final lunge over the top of the hill, and hightailed it to greener pastures.

This near death experience only seemed to whet little Jenny's appetite for horses, and after putting in a few more years learning to stay on at all speeds and in most circumstances, we became the proud young owners of horses of our own. We lived on their backs and in their stalls.

The horses were stabled at Sycamore Farms, a small ranch on Crosscreek Road just a mile or so from our house, under the benevolent eyes of a mountaintop Monastery, whose secretive monks none of us had ever seen.

We could not realize at the time how grand our life was. Ecstatic the day we were given the horses, we quickly began to take it for granted. Didn't most of our friends have horses to compete in the local horseshows, to explore the surrounding hills and valleys, for sunset rides along the beaches? Didn't everyone here have fancy cars, good friends and lovely parents? It seemed so. We were protected, surrounded by every luxury... no one in Malibu seemed to know any other life. Little did I realize this was going to be a hard act to follow.

Our days in Malibu indeed seemed truly out of a fairy tale... loving parents, beautiful golden children, the beach for a sandbox. We thought it normal to live in an oceanfront house with ten bedrooms and a six-car garage, (important to these pages only because one of the occupants, Father's electric blue Talbot racing car, was instrumental in his decision to transplant us all to France).

It seemed normal to have horses stabled within walking distance; a speedboat in front of the house; and the unique "Father touch," a large wooden raft anchored one hundred fifty feet offshore amidst the rolling swells...for sunbathing and water-skiing takeoffs.

Every other year or so, during a particularly rambunctious winter storm, the raft would break loose and sail off to unknown destinations... leaving the turbulent waters and crashing waves wild and unfettered, temporarily free of man's taming influence.

The first calm day of spring, Father would magically show up with another raft, more solid and of larger proportions than the previous. Seals and seagulls displayed their intense enthusiasm at having their offshore resting spot back by offering up piles of droppings...strategically placed to be the first thing we saw or sat on as we pulled ourselves up, gracefully one hoped, out of the water and onto the raft.

The raft was always a great focal point of summer energy. Being visible to the entire Malibu Colony, it attracted both swimmers and water-skiers alike, and was even the venue for impromptu floating barbecues. One calm, perfect water-skiing day a clunky old speedboat pulled up alongside the raft, with a clunky old couple aboard.

"Halloo," they hailed. "Would you mind teaching my wife to waterski?" the old gent asked father. "It looks like so much fun when y'all do it."

"Sure," said Father, eyeing the heavy boat lolling in the water, "My boat or yours?"

"Well, we were sure hoping you could show us with our boat, so we can learn the whole process and ski wherever we are."

"OK," toss me the rope," said Father, gallantly helping the wife onto the raft.

While family and friends spectated (a new word) from various vantage points on our boat and the raft, father instructed the woman, a sweet laughing lady of sixty or so, how to sit on the very edge of the raft for takeoff as we did, how to, "Keep your arms straight in front of you, and above all to let go of the tow rope if you fall."

We always took off from the raft in this manner. With a bit of skill on the part of both skier and boat driver, it was actually possible to stay dry, (often a desirable feat as the Pacific can get pretty cold), assuming you didn't have a splashdown mid-run.

If the takeoff had to be choreographed cleverly, the return to the raft and a waterfree landing was even more delicate. Taking a slow pass by the gently rocking raft, tossing the tow rope aside at just the right time and speed, freesliding towards the raft…then a quick grab at the edge of the raft before you sank and a bit of very precise timing to swing ones buttocks up onto the raft… resulting in theory in a perfectly dry landing, casually sitting on the edge of the raft while the next in line caught the tow line.

Usually this technique was fairly accident free…although heading straight for the raft at a certain speed, upright and without a rope, in swells that were blithely oblivious to the perils they could cause, was always a thrill.

Now it was the elderly lady's turn, and although father would not attempt to let her land back on the raft, she could easily learn to take off from a sitting position on the raft.

"Here y'are," the husband said, throwing Father their version of a ski rope, a weighty old thing better suited to tying up a tanker. Father coiled it thoughtfully, mentally calculating the speed needed for the old boat to obtain liftoff. He carefully placed the tow rope handle in the wife's hands, then dropped the coiled rope on the raft beside her, out of her way.

Father gave the elderly husband the sign to move off at medium speed. We watched in suspense as the coiled rope unwound slowly. The boat was so slow, so heavy in the water, that father gave the sign to "Hit it," with only half the rope unwound.

To both the spectator's and father's amazement, there was a loud roar from the engines of the heavy old boat as it took off at what looked to be a great speed, particularly given the amount of rope still laying patiently on the raft.

The last coil disappeared in a rush, the woman gripping tightly… she was airborne in a flash, never touching the water for twenty feet. She had a bit of a crash landing, then proceeded, quite unconsciously I am sure, to ignore father's good advice about letting go if you fall, and became a human submarine for a good fifty yards.

Perhaps finally hearing the frantic shouts of the audience, "Let Go, Let Go!!" she did just that, resurfacing slowly. Father rushed in his boat to scoop her out of the water sure she was half dead, and brought her swiftly back to the raft… where she threw her arms to the sky and shouted, "That was Great, let's do it again!"

* * * * *

Adjacent to the Big House in Malibu was a second beachfront lot where the shaded stillness of the formal English style garden was interrupted only by riots of unruly rose bushes, stridently calling for attention; "See my beauty, smell my perfume."

Protected from the beach by a high glass wall, this serene setting was unusual even by Malibu standards, and held a deep secret. The garden was the pink topping on the cake, hiding an entrance to the dark exciting center where hidden from prying eyes, in the womb of the garden, lived an underground bomb shelter. Father built the shelter in a time when there was a great possibility one might be needed, in the late fifties, when supposedly sane Heads of State were eager for any excuse to test their red 'Panic Buttons'. The shelter was designed by Father to house and protect a large family comfortably for several months.

For the comfort of the body, the shelter was complete with air filters, special foods, water, lighting, and all the latest survival paraphernalia available at the time. For the mind, there were puzzles, games and reading materials sufficient for the duration of an attack and cooling off period. A space-age periscope was designed to peer out from the safety of the hatch to survey the surroundings in the aftermath; a mechanical eyeball view of whatever might be left of Malibu in the event of a nuclear attack.

When opened from above the ground, the airtight hatch presented a shiny circular slide for quick entry, the slick white sides disappearing into a tight curve into the darkness. A clip from old

TV newsreels appears in the beginning credits of the movie, "Blast from the Past," starring Bendan Frasier. It shows several members of our family lining up to slide down into the bombshelter, and at least three of my brothers and sisters can be seen disappearing down the hatch.

Although its real purpose was never tested, the bomb shelter was a constant source of wonder to the neighborhood children. Jumping down the hatch onto the smooth slide, twisting at high speed into the darkness to be shot out like a cannonball into the black stomach of a twenty-five by eight foot cylinder deep underground… that was a thrill *sans pareil*.

With lights on, the fold-down bunks attached to the sloping walls sprang into view, and on rare occasions the bombshelter became the venue for sleepless slumber parties. The discussions far into the night revolved not only around the impressive air-testing equipment and the best ways to survive a holocaust, but the more important question of whether or not a large family, given to raucous squabbles at the best of times, could survive being cooped up underground together for weeks on end, without resorting to murder and mayhem.

Father sold the lot a few years later to Jascha Heifetz, violinist extraordinaire. When a house was built over the rose garden, the bombshelter became a wine cellar of spectacular dimensions, and once again the talk of the town.

My brothers and sisters all attended Our Lady of Malibu, a storybook school five minutes from the house, nestled in the curve of a hill now shadowed by the sumptuous grounds of Pepperdine College. Lucky students can now enjoy sweeping views of my childhood stomping grounds. Down the hill to the large wooden show ring where we competed in barrel racing and horsemanship trials almost every month, across Pacific Coast Highway to the parallel little Old Malibu Road leading to the homes of the now Rich and Famous. Houses jostling for room on the yellowgray sands of my youth, sumptuous houses from Malibu Pier to the surfing swells of our smiling bay.

Before Pepperdine was built, the hills in summertime were made for horseback riding. Wild mustard plants, "high as an elephant's eye," towered above my sister Jenny and I as our horses wended their way along the paths made by wild deer. At the end of summer, the yellow mustard flowers had dried away to dust and seed, leaving only the tall, dry stalks.

I was still a relatively small shrimp at the end of my tenth summer, weighing in at about eighty pounds and four feet nothing, my sister not much bigger. Riding along single file through the mustard fields, chatting about sisterly things, we couldn't really see anything but the tall stalks, and large abandoned bird's nests cleverly woven between them here and there.

Suddenly at a twist in the trail, my horse stopped dead in his tracks… Jenny's horse bumped into his rear with a surprised snort, to which my horse paid no heed…he was riveted to the spot, staring at a half grown *eagle* standing proud but unsure as to his purpose, not ten feet away, directly in our path.

The horses would not go forward, they would not turn around. Eagle, kids and horses all eyed one another for ten seconds that seemed an eternity. Suddenly spreading out huge wings, the eagle tilted its wicked curved beak directly at us, and lifted off in the only direction clear of the entangling mustard stalks… straight towards my horse, now frantically trying to spin away. Swooping three feet off the ground, the eagle passed at low altitude under the belly of the stunned animal. Chaos ensued. The horses went straight up, we kids went straight down, and the young eagle, having found his purpose, was soaring high above the melee he had wrought. Laughing no doubt.

FROM NEW MEXICO TO MONTE CARLO

How Father became an electronics wizard in California is something I did not pay much attention to, only too happy to indulge in the exciting lifestyle he carved out for us, and so absorbed with my own little world of daily happenings it's a wonder I noticed anything at all.

Soon after moving from England to California, Father's computer designs had caught the eye of a backer, and Benson-Lehner was created in Santa Monica to build his visionary electronic creations. The company grew quickly, with Father's only competition at the time being two other fledgling computer companies, *Friden* and *IBM*.

I have to marvel now at his prescience of the space age and its futuristic demands, ideas that germinated possibly during a stint in White Sands, New Mexico. The nature of his work there was secret, however I do know he became acquainted with a lifelong friend, Wernher von Braun, the German-born scientist described by Grolier's Encyclopedia as; "a driving force in the development of manned space flight, Von Braun directed the development of the rockets that put humans on the moon."

For those of you interested in how known Nazi supporters were recruited for employment by the United States in the aftermath of WWII, *Wikipedia* states the following;

"**Operation Paperclip** was the Office of Strategic Services (OSS) program used to recruit the scientists of Nazi Germany for employment by the United States in the aftermath of World War II (1939–45). It was conducted by the Joint Intelligence Objectives Agency (JIOA), and in the context of the burgeoning Soviet–American Cold War (1945–91); one purpose of *Operation Paperclip* was to deny German scientific knowledge and expertise to the USSR, and the UK.

Although the JIOA's recruitment of German scientists began after the European Allied victory (8 May 1945), US President Harry Truman did not formally order the execution of *Operation Paperclip* until August 1945. Truman's order expressly excluded anyone found "to have been a member of the Nazi Party, and more than a nominal participant in its activities, or an active supporter of Nazi militarism." Said restrictions would have rendered ineligible most of the scientists the JIOA had identified for recruitment, among them rocket scientists Wernher von Braun and Arthur Rudolph, and the physician Hubertus Strughold, each earlier classified as a "menace to the security of the Allied Forces".

To circumvent President Truman's anti-Nazi order, and the Allied Potsdam and Yalta agreements, the JIOA worked independently to create false employment and political biographies for the scientists. The JIOA also expunged from the public record the scientists' Nazi Party memberships and régime affiliations. Once "bleached" of their Nazism, the US Government granted the scientists security clearance to work in the United States. *Paperclip*, the project's operational name, derived from the paperclips used to attach the scientists' new political personae to their "US Government Scientist" JIOA personnel files."

Von Braun and several other top German scientists (aerospace engineers) continued their rocket research at the U.S Airforce White Sands Missile Range …now side by side with British and American scientists.

Wafting across my mind floats a picture of those months in White Sands, New Mexico. High mounds of the purest, whitest, finest sand I have ever encountered in all my subsequent travels. These white mountains return to me as a distant yet vivid memory; mammoth guardians of an endless stretch of rollicking road, straight and narrow, a two-lane blacktop disappearing at the far end of my vision in a hot, shimmering mirage.

It was a storybook road with impossible dips and highs, a rollercoaster road, that made the carload bounce and scream with toddler's laughter as the white mounds flashed by on either side… happy memories of scrambling out of the car to climb an extra high mountain, sliding down the huge piles of warm white sand on a creatively flattened cardboard box, with Father's high tech options; a jutting 'prow' and a rope handle. My small shrieking brother, Christopher, hanging on for dear life, caught up as we tumbled down the bottom of the hill into the arms of laughing young parents.

White Sands. Bits of life stored and remembered at the discretion of my brain, without any consultation from me, determining of its own volition which pictures to keep and which to discard… thus offering me glimpses of hauntingly sad memories just as unexpectedly as happy ones.

This particular memory of laughter and white sands I shall make my own again, adding it to the vignettes of early times stored in a richly adorned gembox tucked in a corner of my mind. This precious memory I'll place carefully on a golden top shelf, to be admired and looked at fondly. The bottom, darker shelf is kept locked.

That these glistening dunes were not made of sand, but rather of powdery white gypsum, the main ingredient in plaster of Paris, is something I read only recently, grateful for the timing of this bittersweet trivia.

White Sands was perhaps the steppingstone for father's computer passion. With his own company established in California, he was now free to focus on peaceful applications for his creativity and inventions. No more acoustic homing torpedoes, navigational bombsights, or heat sensitive missiles, the kind of government projects he found himself involved in during his Air Force days in England, and quite possibly at White Sands. Computers, and the discovery of their myriad applications, became his life.

On weekends he was no longer a serious computer designer. Leaving his computer babies humming safely at the office, the weekends in Malibu were full of adults laughing, chatting, swimming and tossing together fabulous meals on the barbeque, while we kids trekked sand in and out of the house ad nauseum, with never a complaint from Mom. "That's what beach houses are for," she would say with a grin.

From a pale English rosebud, Mom had blossomed in the California sun. Tan, pretty, and busty has always been an unbeatable combination, and there was usually at least one vice-president from father's company following her around to do her bidding; bring a drink, haul a chair, maybe even discuss something serious once in a while.

She had competition though. Father's female assistants were usually attractive, and often visited the house on weekends. Nancy was one who visited us regularly. On good terms with both mother and father, she felt comfortable inviting a blind date to meet her at our house one Saturday afternoon, explaining,

"This way I won't be stuck alone with him if he turns out to be a troll." Father was hit with a 'prank' idea. Engaging the complicity of the entire family, he outlined his plan, and answered the door himself when 'Todd' arrived.

Now we all know that short, balding men can be powerhouses in their own right. Rich ones are often considered attractive and sexy by the most beautiful women… father however, appeared not to have been aware of that. He deemed that this man standing in front of him, with a black patch over one eye to boot, was not what he envisioned for Nancy… or perhaps he was just carried away with the idea of The Prank.

He introduced Todd to his assistant Nancy, saying, I'd like you to meet my wife, Jane." Next he introduced Todd to my attractive, vibrant mother, saying, "And this is your date, Nancy."

Well, watching this poor man call our mother "Nancy", and chatting her up like there was no tomorrow, had us all in stitches. We kids (several of us teenagers by now) calling the real Nancy "Mom," dragged her out of earshot into the kitchen and demanded she make us lunch while we stood by chortling, at which she dissolved on the floor in gales of laughter. Even on our best behavior in Todd's presence, it was impossible to hide the smirks and giggles. He must have thought we were an exceptionally happy family.

Periodically, after a particularly moonish remark to our Mum by Todd, as he knelt at her feet with a glass of wine and looked up at her adoringly, we would dash into another room and stagger around beating the walls with glee, Father was pounding the floor this time with tears of laughter.

For an entire afternoon we called Nancy 'Mom'. For an entire afternoon this poor man courted another man's wife, right in front of us all. I do not remember the exact moment Father finally let him off the hook with the truth. I do know his mortification knew no bounds, and that he flew, never to be seen or heard of again. Todd, we apologize.

* * * * *

I mentioned the Big House in Malibu had a six-car garage. It was a thing of beauty in and of itself, with six individual garage-doors presenting a united front on the Old Malibu Road. An impressive green entrance door opened onto a wide flight of stairs leading down to the gardens, the house and the beach.

A walkway meandered casually through landscaped gardens, seemingly only vaguely intent on reaching the front door. Then "wait a minute, what's this?" A candy striped awning tucked away in a garden alcove catches the eye; an old fashioned Soda Fountain, complete with French café tables and shade umbrellas, designed by Father for his towheaded kids. I cherish an old photo showing three of my little siblings, ages maybe three to six, their spun golden hair wafting in the breeze, perched on intricate ironwork chairs around a fancy little table, sipping sodas under the pink stripes… oblivious to the fact that life didn't get much better than this.

The six garages were home to a variety of residents; a dark brown Lincoln Continental convertible; my metallic blue Chevy, bought upon my return to Malibu after surviving a year in a boarding school in the South of France (where quite providentially I learned a fair amount of French). Then there was my mother's faded old beige DeSoto we called "the Hunchback," of which she was inordinately fond… that she treasured in fact, for her own rebellious reasons.

An English maiden not interested in any forms of snobbism, her late teenage years were sabotaged, like Father's, by WWII. Her earlier childhood was also lost to her when her mother killed herself. The young woman I was never to meet or call Grandmother was consigned to a long stay in a Swiss hospital, a sanatorium I think they were called in those days. As she lay fading away, slowly dying of tuberculosis, her misery and loneliness were compounded by unrequited love for a handsome young doctor, happily married to another. When my Mother was only a little waif of nine, her mother ended her life with the very pills intended to ease her pain.

Which left my mother alone with her dad, a brilliant English inventor, with a temper to match. (Just now realizing that this "temper" was gifted to me by the family genes, will make it easier for me to deal with). One of his most lucrative ideas was something to do with bicycle wheel valves, for which his family may even now receive royalties. Grandfather was also the author of the classic Second World War guide *"Aircraft Recognition"*, published by Penguin Books in 1941, and reprinted in 1990 to coincide with the fiftieth anniversary of the Battle of Britain. His text provided "a definitive catalogue of the airplanes, enemy and friendly, seen over British skies during the Second World War."

Sometime after he was left alone, Grandad married a woman twenty years his junior, my very elegant and lovely step-grandmother. I don't know how things went for my mother during this part of her life, as this is not a subject that has ever been broached between us; how this little girl must have mourned the loss of her mother I cannot even imagine.

It occurs to me now as I write, that while my mother would have been loved and cared for as a little girl by her new stepmother, she could never have known anything even closely resembling our fun and carefree Malibu lifestyle.

I hope this brings my mother pleasure then, to know her children had those few magnificent years. I hope there was love between her and her new mother when she was little; I want to believe it, as I'm not sure I can bear thinking of another sad little childhood like that of my own daughter. Pangs of regret and guilt I cannot shake completely still surface unexpectedly, despite our now rather splendid new life. I do know this elegant English lady presided over her husband's well being for fifty-two or so years until he died at the rich age of ninety three. As well as his temper, I have high hopes of also inheriting his genes relating to longevity.

Monica and Grandad lived atop one of Monte Carlo's earliest and most elegant high-rises, the Palais Heracles. The building sits smack above the Royal Box set up every year in May for the Royal family view the Grand Prix. High up on the fourteenth floor, the building's flowered terraces gaze daily over one of the most beautiful ports in the world. Only Porto Rotondo in Sardinia, and St. Tropez, those tiniest ports with the biggest yachts, come even close to the splendor of this vast port. The Monte Carlo municipal swimming pool sparkles below Grandad's penthouse, flanked on the right by Rainier's Grimaldi Palace, and on the left by the curving hillside upon which the Hotel de Paris perches in all its majesty.

The Port of Monte Carlo is home to many of the most beautiful yachts on the seven seas. During the Grand Prix in May every year, the bay turns into a white tapestry of boats lazing side by side, from the base of Rainier's palace to the sweep of hill winding up to the Casino.

For many summers after the move from California to France, which you will hear about in detail before long, the Grand Prix drew me, along with thousands of others, to its throbbing noisy rapturous heart. A week of trial races and noise, hot cars and hotter drivers, their beautiful girlfriends and frantic groupies, TV cameras, parties… a wild week in this usually subdued and elegant town, a crazy week right up to the day of reckoning, the race itself; which I need not describe here as it is televised every year in all its glory.

Monegasque policemen in their handsome uniforms grinned charmingly as they lifted me over barriers that block off the street for this entire chaotic week. Barricades that necessitated just such extreme measures to reach Monaco's popular portside swimming pool, shimmering invitingly just beyond the bleachers lining the main road. I probably could have made it by myself over the barriers to the crystal pool we preferred to the stony beaches, however why pass up those glowing moments, with enthusiastic help so readily available?

Chatting with Mario Andretti (Senior) while he knelt by his right front tire checking something mysterious and mechanical before a practice run, is still a fond memory. Somewhere I have photos that show it was not only my scintillating conversation that was holding his interest; Mario is looking up, right up it appears, under the short, braless, tanktop I was wearing. The top covered me well enough from normal angles, but was not designed for ground-to-boob peeking.

I loved visiting my grandparents, they were so formal, so *British*. We used to tiptoe around them when we were youngsters, terrified of upsetting Grandad who was known to holler and stomp…yet he could be a good sport, often taking large groups of us water-skiing on his ChrisCraft with the beautifully polished wood trim, or out to dinner at night, where he was the king of that understated British humor. Still, he terrified us.

My lovely granny admitted a secret to me a few years before Granddad's death. "In all my married life," she said, "one of the things I often long for is to have enough time to myself to soak undisturbed in a hot tub of bubbles, with a French pâté sandwich and a glass of champagne." Apparently this was unthinkable while her 'proper' British husband was alive, needing her at once, and at any moment…Granny, may you now soak and sandwich in blissful solitude.

This parental structure no doubt had much to do with my own mother's basic unflappable nature, and her refusal to take seriously my "Code of Important Things in the Life of a Teenager."

Shortly before I was shipped out of Malibu to a boarding school in England, my mind still holds one unpleasant picture of me as a fearful teenager, standing on the brick steps of Marymount High School in Beverly Hills, watching with trepidation as the cars filed up the narrow driveway… Mercedes, Rolls, Lincolns all rolled up with quietly humming engines to collect their little darlings. No BMW's or fancy SUV's in vogue yet, was there really ever such a time?

I remember praying intently that Mother wouldn't embarrass me by showing up in her beat up old DeSoto, even pleaded to Anyone listening Up There that she would have the sense to pick me up in the Lincoln. I am now pleased to note that God had better things to do with His time than listen to my petty whining. He never paid any attention to my selfish wishes at all, and of course mother often showed up with her Hunchback… and I survived. Yet even at that age I was mindful that admiration and respect are tendered instinctively to men and women driving expensive cars...the old adage, "Don't judge a book by it's cover," be damned.

Marymount, in spite of its reputation at the time for academic excellence, was the reason for my long standing feud with Catholicism in general, and recitation of the Rosary in particular. The nuns required a specific number of Hail Marys to be said per day by all students. Honoring this stipulation was effected by ordering us to say out loud as many prayers as we could fit in while changing hurriedly into our gym clothes; there we were, scrabbling over locker space, hopping on one foot and then another to get into the blasted gym shorts in the cramped space, rushing to be on time, all the while trying to recite our Hail Marys.

While this may have been a brilliant tactic on the part of the nuns to quell teenage gossip and giggles, it struck me as a particularly unspiritual way to say prayers, and introduced a skepticism concerning the Catholic belief system in general that stuck with me for years.

Once the school was behind me, I found in fact it had put me right off prayer altogether, leaving me traipsing around different countries for several years, rudderless, in and out of precarious situations, with no one on my side that I was aware of... until I began flying. At night, alone.

It did not matter what country I was living in, what job I had, nor what lifestyle I was living, the denouement was always the same: climbing to the highest pinnacle available in my dream state, I had no fear of diving out into the abyss, arms outstretched, face forward, body gliding downward smoothly, the wind in my face. Sheer aerodynamic bliss for five seconds. Then the rapid descent, and the earth rushing up to meet me.

Despite all efforts to stop the downward flight, despite my strenuous, Herculean struggle to soar back up to the heights, my body plummeted towards the ground like a diving falcon intent on lunch; arms now tight against my sides, wind so harsh in my face I could barely see. A rapid, facefirst descent to an altitude so low that chest and stomach brushed the treetops, then the tops of lower plants and bushes, until finally I am skimming along inches off the earth's surface, still in fast forward movement, still face downward... seeing every particle of earth flying by just under my nose, mind and body locked in a desperate struggle to turn upwards again, to raise my body higher, (to a higher level?) to avoid the inevitable crash.

Milliseconds before my tense body ground into the earth, I would awake, sweat pouring off me from my exertions, the question still ringing in my ears, "Why couldn't I fly?"

Ten years of this dream, two or three times annually, the only variation being the pinnacles found for the jump-off, and the different landscapes I struggled to gain altitude over... desserts, mountains, fields...strangely, or perhaps luckily, never lakes or oceans. For ten years the ending was always the same; face to face with the earth... before awaking startled, exhausted and troubled.

For no reason I can pinpoint, one night it happened. Swan diving off a high, green mountaintop, the beginning was perfect as always, peaceful, beautiful...and then the dreaded descent. Desperately I asked of no-one in particular, "What do I have to do to Fly!?"

Instantaneously my mind began reciting The Lord's Prayer, hidden in the folds of my subconscious since those early days in Catholic School. (I notice now with a smile as I write, that it was *not* the Hail Mary). With a graceful swoop, my flight direction changed like that of a roller coaster going from steep downward roll, into graceful ascent.

Up and up I soared, leveled off and FLEW. I flew over rich valleys, over houses and mountains, I could see everything from my eagle's eye perspective. I could turn right, I could turn left, I could swoop and climb, roll and twist, no longer bound by the forces of past plummeting descents. I could see everything far below me with an indescribable clarity…I could fly!

I awoke refreshed, happy thrilled, and with a healthy respect for prayer again. I have not had the dream since.

GRUNION HUNTS AND MALIBU FOREST FIRES

As these pages develop, I am often asked whether I have an 'outline' for the book. Seeing my quiet, peaceful lifestyle on our secret island in the Bahamas, people I meet seem compelled to ask *"but what do you do?!"* My flip reply is "as little as possible," which incurs a startled, somewhat jealous laugh.

If I deem they are entitled to a bit more data, yet I have no wish to reveal the financial synopsis of my life; ie the management crises dealt with, the deals negotiated, the real-estate opportunities grasped, the hours of late night number crunching… plus the plain good luck, and many blessings that have brought me to this place in my life, I offer that I am occupied with writing. This often leads to the outline question.

I'm sure I should have an outline, everyone seems to think so. However the answer is No. These pages were begun without any thought of a book. My daughter walked out the door… distraught, my body walked to the computer, and my hands began to type. The first five pages wrote themselves.

Thoughts come rolling out as they please. Recollections jump into my mind at the oddest moments, often I am forced to grope around for pen and paper at three in the morning… eyes unwilling to focus, yet the brain urgently insisting I act as its scribe. In the morning the writing is difficult to decipher, yet usually amazing in the detail and depth of what has poured out while I, as my body, was pretty much asleep.

The trick is to put these voluminous notes in felicitous order. To assure they flow not whimsically here and there, but show signs of vigorous intent, a spirited determination to squire us with wit and candor through a 'beginning, middle and end'… apparently other essential items a writer should not be seen without.

Note added during post production of Honey English: Mark Twain's editors released his autobiography in 2010, 100 years after his death, as he requested. He desired the freedom to write with the knowledge that anyone he put in his pages would not be alive to be adversely affected. A noble thought, however one that by his documented struggles, did not make writing his memoirs any easier for him.

I am convulsed with laughter now reading that over one hundred years ago Mark Twain also grappled with the 'beginning, middle and end' dilemma of his memoirs, coming to the same conclusion I did… or vice versa; that an autobiography is a living thing and as such must be compelling and vibrant. It must encompass past reminiscences and current thoughts fresh from the brain… in whichever order they tumble… 'beginning, middle and end' be damned. Thank you Mark Twain for your timely 100 year old support of my theory.

I do not consider myself a writer. The word itself invokes the thought of someone who has actually been published. Someone to be admired not only for the hours they have spent writing, but for summoning the strength to plow through the next phase of finding a publisher who thinks the pages are worth putting in print. That to me is a writer. I see myself as someone who is just 'writing', just getting interesting bits of life on paper, my very own True Adventure. If the rest follows, it will be a lovely miracle.

The idea of a 'book' only began to flit around my head as the pages continued to flow, albeit erratically, and not at all in the disciplined, orderly way one hears is the acceptable method of writing. Rather, several weeks at a time would pass without my wanting to even look at the last pages written. Then a sudden frenzy of creativity. Thus an outline still seems unlikely.

This writing is taking me I know not where. Going with the wind and a prayer, no guidelines, except keeping an eye out whenever possible for deference to the sensitivities of the English language. We will know where we are when we get there.

Thus I allow myself a bit of leeway on the rules, trusting it will all work out, and that this elucidation to you will envelop any blips or unsmooth transitions from one country to another, or one subject to another as the pages unfold.

Working with a Gemini mind, (a hop and a skip, butterfly kind of mind), you and I are exploring and discovering together. At this very moment, a goal… not an outline, but a superb goal, has bubbled up from the depths of this blended creativity.

'To enthrall, to amuse, to captivate with a well turned phrase, to invoke one's passion for our story.' That is a rainbow of a goal, and like the elusive rainbow, the beauty is to be reveled in, sought after, beheld in the mind's eye. A worthy goal, and sufficient for me just now.

Still waiting for that wicked imp of mine to come home. At what point do I stop waiting, stop fretting, and just go and find my lovely, rude girl? Not yet, I know she is not in danger, just angry. She will not be glad to see me if I find her, will not want to come home with me…this is not a question of her safety, rather my desire to set things right; so there is no point instigating a public battle of wills in front of her friends.

I will wait and write a bit longer, time to let her come home by herself. I'll bide the time with recollections destined to amuse and lift the spirit… we'll drift back to the carefree years when the most important event on the agenda was a prospective Grunion Hunt, the treasured Grunion Hunt.

Since leaving Malibu, there have been only two people in my travels who knew what the phrase, "The Grunion Are Running!" means. It amazes me how a phenomenon so integral to our life in Malibu could be almost totally unknown to the rest of the world.

Grunion are those small, tasty, anchovy-like fish that swim in schools at night off the gently sloping beaches of Southern California during their spawning season. Mother Grunion are mysterious and wonderful creatures, waiting for just the right wave to bring them in to lay their eggs. Not just any old wave, nor any old night will do, as proven by many fruitless nights we spent as supervised youngsters, and later as unsupervised teenagers, huddled on the beach in blankets waiting in vain for the first trumpeting cry, "The Grunion are Running!" The signal to roll out of the blankets and bring home the breakfast.

No, not just any wave or any night; the Grunion window of opportunity is brief… only the *"first four nights after the highest tide of the full moon, or the new moon"* will do. A bit of accurate trivia I share with you from Grolier's Multimedia Encyclopedia.

Technically, Grunion don't 'run' at all. Calculating the moon and the tides with the precision of a drill sergeant, thousands of female fish *surf* in on their chosen wave, crashing onto the shoreline in a wriggling mass. As the froth recedes, the beach becomes a glittering, slithering mass of female grunion *dancing on their tails…* yes, standing upright and digging frantically into the wet sand to lay their eggs, while the males roll around doing the Fertilizing Quickstep. Within twenty-five seconds, or the time it takes the next wave to roll in and wash them out, each female will lay close to 2000 eggs.

It is near midnight and the beach is alive with the long awaited cries, "The Grunion are here, the grunion are running!" Children, teenagers, parents, race up and down the dark beach with buckets and flashlights. Despite admiration for the noble attempts of the grunion to procreate in this odd fashion, the passion of the hunt coupled with culinary desire overcomes the masses.

Eco talk and environmental protection are a speck in the future; this is the late sixties, and breakfast is caught in what has to be the most ungainly manner. When mere hands prove too cumbersome and failure to catch the slippery delicacy becomes a mean reality, the method of choice for many is to cast all inhibitions aside, throw oneself bodily onto a wave of wriggling silver, flattening all in reach with the stomach, imprisoning the catch, hands groping, arms and feet flailing, scooping. Then the getaway. Clutching the wriggling prize, dashing to higher ground before the next wave crashes over fisher and fishee alike.

The timing has to be split-second perfect. Too soon, and a facefull of water is your only reward - too late and the next breaker rolls in, leaving the hapless hunter buried under crashing waves and frantic female fish eager to deposit their eggs and cut ties with offspring they will never see.

Shrieks of delight up and down the beach carry on late into the night, the cries dying down only when the Grunion disappear as mysteriously as they arrived. Deciding this is not the peaceful egg-laying ground they envisioned, they glide *en masse* down the coast to a more lonely stretch of beach. Dedicated surfers looking for the perfect wave.

Our Grunion Hunts were sheer midnight lunacy, shared by mad stalkers of small fish. An acceptable excuse for teenagers to cuddle in blankets, listening intently for that first gleeful shout, the signal the sea has deigned to deposit her silver bounty at our feet. A strange myth to many, a reality only to those who have happily crunched the crispy fried fish whole the next morning, and remember forever the taste, the laughter and the magic.

It was during this carefree time, while our airlift to a new life in the French countryside was only the seed of an idea germinating in Father's busy brain, that a fire threatened to rip our lives apart. One of the devastating Los Angeles fires that are hypnotizing to watch safely on television… a different story altogether when your life, family, home, possessions and pets are directly in its path.

The fires always started at night. At the end of summer, Malibu residents are ever alert to the arrival of the Santa Ana winds. Teasingly warm at first, an 'Indian Summer' in late November, it is impossible to enjoy their light caress, as they are but a harbinger of the heat and madness to come.

Winds with a twisted mind of their own that soon tire of drying the chaparral to a crackling mass of sticks. Joining forces, the winds begin their hot, provocative dances through the canyons and hills, inviting covert pyromaniacs to dance with them…enticing them, seducing them… until the first match is offered and the blaze begins.

For the next few days and late into the nights, vigilant neighbors discuss wind velocity, they calculate timing, they plan strategies, they ask vital questions; how much time do we have left, how far away are the flames, what new heights have they reached, how fast are they moving?

Each family is weighing their nefarious choices; to risk all with a last minute escape, or prudently leave while the fire is still several miles away, sparing life and loved ones, but very likely losing the house. By day three the ashes are thick and heavy, a swirling, flurrying, gray suffocating snow.

The hard core... the stupid, the brave, the stubborn, the fighters, my father among them, choose to save the houses. Perched precariously high on the rooftops, armed with woefully inadequate hoses, resolutely they wet down the buildings, keeping a watchful eye on the advancing flames.

The fire is relentless. Every minute now the rooftop heroes reevaluate the speed of the marching wall of flame, note every gyration of the wind. Every sapbursting explosion clones a new set of flaming soldiers, marching closer, closer. The cars on the road below are at the ready; children, pets, valuables packed... mothers poised to flee at the last possible moment.

We teenagers, (barely qualifying at ages eleven and thirteen) have a job to do now; rescue the horses from the ranch hidden in the narrow strip of Crosscreek Road, not far - not far at all, from the advancing army of fire.

Thus my sister Jenny and I find ourselves dropped off by a neighbor at the ranch in the dark of night, in the middle of a blistering hot gale, trying to saddle up frantic horses at midnight. When the smell of smoke becomes overwhelming and the horses beyond calming, we give up on the saddles and throw ourselves on bareback.

The only way out of the canyon is to ride the terrified horses along Crosscreek Road to the comparative safety of the beach. This one-lane, bumpy, twisty, rutted, scenic unpaved loop dives off, then back onto the Pacific Coast Highway. It is named for the concrete crossing that fords the creek where it runs past the ranch.

My childhood name for this lively stream was Raindaughter. After passing leisurely through the San Fernando Valley, she picks up speed and races along a deep, narrow gulch the length of Malibu Canyon. Finally bursting out of the confines of the canyon, the water spills and spreads, and there Raindaughter dallies for a while, resting, at the base of the canyon wall.

Gathering strength, she swirls and pulses into a deep, sandfringed waterhole, creating a cool oasis with a tiny beach on one side. High slate boulders on the other side sprout a magically placed overhanging tree adorned with the alltime kid pleaser, Tarzan's rope.

How many times we kids grabbed, flew, dropped into that cool murky water…how many times did we just miss the deadly watermoccasin I saw with my own eyes on a later, adult visit. Black evil eyes and forked tongue barely raising a ripple, gliding silently in the water under the frayed old rope, he was sharing the shade of our childhood swimming pool.

Satisfied with her landscaping efforts, Raindaughter leaves the welcoming pool she has created and heads briskly towards the ranch. At the 'crossing' the narrow road takes a rather treacherous dip down into the stream, the water skims across a wide concrete slab, until the road heads steeply up the other side.

In winter and spring the little river is very busy; spilling over the thick concrete in a baby waterfall, then trundling happily alongside the road to its intersection with Pacific Coast Highway a half mile away. Skipping and singing, she rarely varies her chosen route, kissing the little road goodbye only in time to veer off and dip beneath the highway bridge. Merging briefly with the lagoon near the Malibu Pier, she races joyously across the last sand dune between herself and her destiny, the Pacific Ocean.

During stormy weather and heavy rains, my dancing Raindaughter has been known to show her might and render the crossing impassible.

Oftimes forceful and aggressive, she can also be coy and moody, thin and lively, heavy and lazy… her moods swinging wider with the changing seasons than a provocative woman's.

Now at summer's end Raindaughter is but a shadow of herself, trickling along in shallow rivulets, barely keeping the riverstones wet, the bigger ones lying exposed and parched in the daytime sun. Just lazing along, sulking now, her lover the ocean is the last thing on her mind. Torpid, tame, weak… bankrupt of protection from the flames soon to pour down the tortuous canyon. This depleted little summer stream offers no refuge from the fire on this wild and crazy night.

Bareback on fretting horses, leading two others, Jenny and I head out into the murky darkness along the edge of Crosscreek Road, searching for the path that is so easy to ride in daylight, so easy to see as it ducks under the highway right beside the sulky stream.

The horses are righteously skittish, the path barely visible, the going slow and tense. Not enough hands for flashlights. What we need now is light. Suddenly an eruption blinds us. Giant flamethrowers have topped the mountain to the north and just beyond our house, shooting orange rockets into the sky along the length of a mile long crest. Now we have light… too much light. Too late to be careful what one wishes for.

Awe, fear, terror, those are boring, overused words. Not good enough. Where is the language to describe the thunder of our young hearts? Quieting the stomping horses, the lighting now more than adequate, we make for the beach at a brisk trot, pass under the bridge and head straight into the sea, until the water reaches the horses' shoulders.

The horses are tossing and splashing now, unhappy with this miserable selection of choices; death by fire or death by the rolling sea. As we urge them towards the house a mile up the beach, each new burst of flame on the mountaintop competes with the last in height and intensity, showering us with bits of burning branches and debris. Not to be outdone, the wind descends from the mountains, claws at our clothes, howls in our faces, force-feeding us a grimy diet of ash and soot.

Over my shoulder Jenny's fear is reflected in the orange light of the flames. Tears streaming down her face, desperately struggling to maintain her balance on the slippery back of her wet and thrashing horse, holding the mane and reins tight in one hand, she leans against a sodden neck, gently encouraging the wild eyed horses on the leadlines to follow us. A brave little girl in a nightmare… on a mare in the night.

What a rush of relief as we spot Father atop the roof, silhouetted by the flames leaping over the last hill separating house from fire. The thrill is shortlived, the fire is too close. One man against this fiery world. What gives him the strength, the passion to do battle with Nature's fire-breathing dragons, hammered with the knowledge that fire trucks and their professionally trained men have withdrawn to a safer distance?

A rooftop neighbor screams the news to us that Mother was forced to flee with her car-full of precious baggage, bowing to pressure to evacuate from the exhausted firemen. Soaking wet, horses shivering from fear, we watch helplessly from the sea as the wall of flame races mouth wide open down the hill, hell bent on devouring the last barrier before the house... The Old Malibu Road.

A minuscule strip of asphalt two cars wide, it was a tiny joke of a road then. No 'through traffic' allowed, it was useful only to residents visiting friends, or going home. It heaved where huge tree roots twisted under it, caved where the sea bashed it. A vulnerable little road. All that was left had between our house and the fire.

A lightweight jump for those taunting, exuberant flames, impatiently demanding now only one rush of capricious wind. And capricious the wind was, changing direction just as the flames licked the very edges of the road, forcing them angrily back over already blackened, bare land. Was it possible? Were the flames truly retreating, defeated in the end by their own Mother Nature? Or is this a cruel trick. Are they toying with us, with our destiny? Hearts in mouths we watched, we waited.

That I am here to tell the tale is all the answer you need; in the early gray dawn the fire gave up, betrayed by the changing winds gleefully racing back across the smoldering landscape to assess the homeless wildlife. Deer, skunks and the occasional puma with blackened feet and singed fur, those were the few survivors. Bambi's worst nightmare come to life.

OF CASTLES AND CRO MAGNONS

Continuing the rundown on the six garages, safe one more year from the onslaught of forest fires, the fourth one was used for storage, the fifth housed a shiny black Talbot Touring Car, and the sixth garage held father's prize, an outrageously elegant European racing machine. Long, low-slung, impossibly sleek and powerful, this shiny blue Talbot had the misfortune to blow its gearbox twenty-three hours into France's 24 Hour Le Mans race sometime in the fifties. The French driver, Pierre LeVecque, had faultlessly worked the 'preselect' Wilson gearbox (for those in the know) for twenty-three hours, refusing to be relieved by another driver. In the twenty-fourth hour he made an irretrievable shifting error, and the transmission exploded.

When father saw the car and fell in love, it had been repaired and retired from racing. I don't remember if he found it in France or California, but it was a star in either country. The Talbot was Electric Blue, with an open cockpit and lacking many of the basic amenities of an average Street car. No windows, no doors, Father would leap over the side just like any race driver, part of the integral thrill of driving this monster regularly to his Santa Monica office. No windshield wipers, no turn signals, no noticeable muffler. The color and rocket takeoff noise screamed to every passing police car "Stop Me, Stop Me!" And stop him they did.

Cops would walk slowly around the car in disbelief, while the Talbot quivered and frettet, keeping up a low pitched roar in anticipation of being set free again.

Today's cop is a motorcycle cop, resplendent in his California Highway Patrol uniform, dark aviator shades reflecting the electric blue of the Talbot. He is calm and menacing as he approaches the car.

"Turn the engine off," he shouts to father over the impatient throaty rumblings.

With much mime and gesticulation father makes it clear the cop will have to help with a pushstart if the engine were turned off... key ignitions not being featured on European racecars of the fifties.

Still cool but obviously disgruntled, the cop tries again in a loud voice, "Where are the turn signals?" Father flaps his arm left, flaps his arm right and shouts "This is the way they teach it in driving school," oblivious to, or perhaps relishing the sweat breaking out on the cop's face.

"Windshield wipers?" the cop yells in desperation.

"Do they have to be automatic?" Father shouts innocently. Puzzled and wary, the cop mutters, "No" under his breath... Father gleefully swipes his hand back and forth over the tiny five-inch high face guard.

The cop is usually apoplectic by now, the rare ones with a sense of humor would be laughing outright. Although they rarely ticketed him, Father wearied of the game one day, and decided we should live in a country more tolerant, and even welcoming, of persons with his enormous imagination and energy. A place where regulations infringed less on ones private life, where father would not pay seventy percent of his annual income to the government in tax, only to be told how to live his life and drive his cars.

We would go to a country of romance and delicious food, creative people and stunning landscapes… it had to be France, birthplace of father's mum, and his favorite race car… and to a Chateau no less. Yes, father had his heart set on a medieval castle, and nothing else would do.

How would you locate the perfect French abode to suit a feisty large family accustomed to the California ways of life?

If you were my father, you would spend a month with a flamboyant Russian friend, Tolmatchoff, flying a small plane over the most beautiful areas of France, marking on an aerial map each Castle and Manoir that caught your eye from the sky.

Next you would spend an entire summer with this same mad Russian, driving from one castle to the next to see which of these properties spotted from the air might happen to be for sale; which one might be large enough, airy and magnificent enough, comfortable enough… surrounded by such spectacular views and valleys, streams and wildlife… as to quash any qualms a family might have about leaving their perfect life in California.

Father found his dream castle, complete with sixteenth century stained glass windows, a circular 'Astrologer's room' at the top of a tall tower with the twelve Zodiac signs inlaid in a circle on the stone floor. A legendary secret tunnel connected the courtyard well to another castle across the valley.

Standing sixty feet tall, high on a hilltop dominating the valleys and rivers in all directions, Chateau de Chaban's huge sunny bedrooms faced west to catch every last ray of sun, before that blazing globe of fire morphed each summer evening into a peaceful pink glow, disappearing in a sudden flash behind a sister mountain crest a mile away... just in time for the shadows to come out to play... creeping across Chaban's four stories of history sometimes as late as nine p.m. on a Midsummer's Night.

Stone walls five feet thick, impervious to enemy attacks for hundreds of years, laughingly fending off the only enemy now, Mother Nature, whose fiercest summer storms and winter gales are wasted on Chaban's stoic strength.

A place of mystery and architectural miracles, of strength and majesty, of laughter and finally tears...its forty rooms a thrill to wander, a navigational challenge from top to bottom; ballroom, library, formal dining room, living room, ten bedrooms, the tower astrology room, two kitchens... most of the rooms were blessed with intricately woven herringbone parquet floors and striking stone fireplaces, many of them six feet high and just as wide.

Antique benches placed *inside* the huge fireplaces were very popular throughout most of the winter... until father came up with his own take on castle central heating; the electric blanket.

Wine cellar, studio, office, photo lab, five unused rooms in the huge attic, laundry rooms, pantries...and eight bathrooms of a fairly recent vintage... although number nine, the one in the library, was an original.

Hidden by a beautifully carved wooden door that lead apparently, nowhere, the striking antique door concealed a small stone room suspended beyond the outer walls of the library, directly over the gardens. Inside this mysterious cubicle was a built-in stone seat, with an open shaft dropping directly to the gardens three stories below. A Medieval toilet was the only possible explanation. The mystery we didn't solve is what signal was used to warn persons in the garden two floors below... when this excellent throne was in use?

Father's castle was sitting on a thousand acres of wooded hills teaming with deer, pheasant and wild boar, in a part of France so beautiful the Cro-Magnon Man had the good sense to make it his home a couple of million years ago.

An excellent crafter of finely tuned Stone Age tools, and author of stunning cave art preserved in the Grottes de Lascaux ten minutes away. Cro-Magnons and their works are commemorated by a hulking, three-story stone carving of the good man himself, standing in the medieval village of Les Eyzies, just fifteen minutes from Le Moustier; our 'one church, one hotel, one bakery village' nestled at the base of the twisty little mountain road that leads up to the castle.

Sometimes this hulking statue is known as the Mousterian Man, other times the Cro-Magnon Man. It matters not how you address him, for he is not paying attention. Standing guard continuously over his picturesque town, his gaze is fixed longingly across the hills and river towards the cliffs of La Roque St. Christophe; five stories of Prehistoric cave dwellings where no doubt he and his friends spent many a long night around the campfires discussing hunting and women... and perhaps dreaming of beer.

Spread across the estate of Chateau de Chaban were several wine producing vineyards, and a dozen or so stone houses in various stages of disrepair... until father and a French architect turned them into a triumphant blend of modern space and light on the inside, without losing one iota of the charm of the ancient stone walls on the outside.

Father often told us that one day his children would each own one of these beautiful houses.

The Tibetan Lamas came to live with us several years later, initially at the castle, then in a stone farm building converted to a 'Tibetan Center' about a mile away. Father walked back to Chaban in a high good mood one day after a visit with the head Lama, and announced gleefully;

"Isn't this exciting, I've just donated the entire estate to the Lamas!" In the ensuing stunned silence, I would have to remind him of his promise to give each of his children a house. Characteristically, he slapped his thigh and said without a bit of embarassment, "By Jove you're right, I'll have to go and tell them," and dashed off on the spot, down the hillside to their neighboring lodgings, to do just that.

* * * * *

Father did not always look like a mad English scientist. He could also be incredibly dashing, particularly in the black cape and top hat he donned on more than one occasion. At the opening of the Musical adapted from his book, The Peace Book, presented at the Albert Hall in London, and later at the Gala Presentation of the book, December 1982 at the Kennedy Center in Washington, D.C. starring Susannah York as the Storyteller, with an international cast of more than one hundred children acting out his story... he was nothing less than magnificent.

Another cape occasion involved a horse drawn carriage on the Champs Elysees in Paris, a beautiful red-headed young woman (who also happened to be my roommate), Springtime in Paris, and love in the air... a story that has to wait until I have found a way to fit in the very unpleasant divorce of my parents.

At what point Father and Mother's breakup began is hard to pinpoint, but I remember at age thirteen or fourteen, during our beautiful days in Malibu and just before being shipped off to boarding school in England, being put in the awkward position of telling mother "please don't bring your boyfriend into the house again, it's not fair to the smaller kids, you must be more discreet". I did not want my younger brothers and sisters to find a strange man in the house with her as I had, both in various stages of disarray, and remember thinking, *"Father should know, he should do something about it, someone should tell him,"* but it wouldn't be me.

Whether father was having an affair with his pretty secretary as people hinted to me later, I couldn't say. He was attractive and charismatic, both men and women finding him a charming and exciting conversationalist. I know he loved most of his children very much most of the time, and showed it often by organizing amazing family outings. He and Mother included the kids in parties and activities, taking us along on trips when it would undoubtedly have been easier, and far more relaxing, to take a real vacation just the two of them.

Whether he was cheating, and mother was retaliating, I don't know; but if he was, it was not obvious to me, and therein lay the difference. This was a rough time for me in Malibu. I was embroiled in Mother's infidelities, yet not allowed to spend time with my favorite girlfriend just a few doors down in the road. Sarah was two years older than me. She had a boyfriend, she was tall, pretty and wore makeup, and therefore was a possible 'bad influence." I was not to go to her house; she was not to visit me.

The injustice of this tormented me, and I convinced myself that since mother was not acting in a straightforward manner, she could not expect me to abide by her unacceptable rules; I of course continued to see Sarah, albeit in secret.

So the day came when I was in my fourteenth year, skipping back home one afternoon after a visit with Sarah, just thinking girly things about Sarah's room; it was so amazing… airy and light like my own, overlooking the water like my own… but hers had a secret staircase leading up to it, with an invisible door hidden in the wood paneling of the hall. This made it a secret room, a girls-only room. Sitting in the benchseat of the bay windows over the ocean was like being on a boat heading out to sea.

Happy and unsuspecting, imagine my surprise at finding both parents waiting for me outside the front door. In a united front they asked none too kindly, "Where have you been?"

Fear and wariness were my immediate reactions. My body knew trouble was brewing and started to freeze, going into paralysis without my willing or wanting it. There was no time to formulate a lie, and my mouth seemed to be working fine, as evidenced by the truth that burbled out; "Down the road at Sarah's," I said quietly…

My mother's hand lashed out and crashed into my face. Tears sprang to my eyes. I was stunned, but looked at her squarely and said, "That's not fair." I said nothing else… we just stood there, glaring at one another. Sensing there was more to this than the words, father put his face close to mine and gritted between clenched teeth, "What did you mean by that?"

"I can't tell you," I muttered, my knees actually beginning to quake, to move on their own in fear, but my feet stayed planted. Father lunged then, grabbing me by my hair to drag me kicking and screaming up the stairs into my room. Slamming the door he shouted, "Now tell me." When I said nothing he dropped me to the floor, shouting again,

"Tell me what you know about your mother!" Met with my grim silence, he went into a blind rage, eyes popping, spit flying, fists hammering. I don't remember any pain, just the terror.

Between flying fists I shouted, "I can't tell you, mom is standing outside the door listening, she'll kill me!" That got his attention. Staggering up off the floor, he growled, "Don't be so bloody stupid," and flung open the door.

His shock at seeing her standing there, breathing hard against the doorjamb, saying nothing, should have been my sweet revenge. Instead I will carry to my grave the image of my mother…frozen at the door, eyes blazing hatred, not at my father, but boring into my face, into my soul.

Father left me crumpled on the floor, took my mother's arm and left the room. Mother took to her bed soon thereafter… father said it was my fault she was ill. Within a month I was shipped off to the boarding school in England I may have mentioned earlier.

Somewhere…upon exposure to truly inappropriate behavior by our guardians in this life, somewhere between the polar extremities of brooding injustice, cheerful acceptance, or outright denial… somewhere there must be a piece missing.

Given the many chances of coming across imperfect role models or bad experiences during our turbulent travels from youngster to adulthood, it is puzzling that while a safety kit of good judgment, common sense, and spiritual wisdom is touted to be buried somewhere deep inside each of us… this is not accessible to rescue us when we desperately need refuge from the long term effects of childhood traumas. It is nowhere to be found until it is too late…long after Fear and Blame overtake us, leaving us twisting in the wind for years.

This event which has stayed so vividly in my memory may have been only a blip on the horizon for my father, he might not even remember it had I ever asked him. As the years went on, he evolved into a great lover of peace, writing and illustrating The Peace Book in the beautiful surroundings of his hilltop castle office. With a kaleidoscope of sun colors streaming through the stained glass windows, he created a classic that was read by His Holiness Pope Paul II, Anwar el Sadat and Gerald G. Jampolsky M.D., author of Letting Go of Fear. These three men of peace wrote the testimonials printed on the cover of The Peace Book.

The book tells the story of a Russian and American child who become friends. Thinking and searching together they find a way to bring friendship to their two countries. This book about children finding the way to world peace was published in the Reagan, Cold War era. Despite it being kept rather quiet in the publishing world, despite its timing… or because of it, the book has become a classic.

Peace Child International was founded based on The Peace Book, the story was turned into musicals performed by talented children dancing and singing to much acclaim around the world. The first performance was given in London's Royal Albert Hall with Susannah York as the Storyteller, and music by David Gordon, Cat Steven's brother. David Woollcombe wrote and directed the UK and USA Peace Child premieres at the Royal Albert Hall and Kennedy Centre which Rosey Simonds co-produced. They have run Peace Child International together for the past 28 years.

"Peace Child International's mission is to empower young people to BE the change they want to SEE in the world. This theme is at the forefront of each of their projects and programs, and is the standard by which they work. PCI supports young people around the world to produce books, musicals, educational materials, workshops and training courses on their major generational challenges: climate change, peace, human rights, poverty, and sustainable development. PCI also funds young people to undertake community-based action projects of their own through the "Be the Change!" program, and hosts the bi-annual World and European Youth Congress series.

Peace Child International is registered in the UK as an educational charity, and since its founding in 1981 has grown to unite more than 1,500 affiliate groups and networks in over 180 countries."

BANISHED AND BELEAGUERED

The English boarding school to which I was banished turned out to be quite a beautiful place in Sussex, with a lovely white haired, exquisitely prissy Headmistress. I'm afraid I made her life a bit hectic. She was used to ruling with an iron hand, but some of her rules were just made to be broken.

We boarders were not allowed to wash our own hair; *every three weeks* we were marched into the nurse's office, one hundred of us, three at a time, and the nurses would run some shampoo over our heads, barely rinsing it off. The punishment, should we be caught washing our hair between the nurse visits, was to have some disgustingly smelly oil poured over our heads, to remain there until the next scheduled washing time. It was a risk we all felt was worth taking, and wet-haired girls crept stealthily around the halls at the oddest times of night to avoid the prying nurses.

It has never been made clear to me whether this impossible rule was to save water, or to assure no one caught cold running around the draughty school halls with wet hair… or just to annoy us. Whatever the reason, no one could live with it, and there were girls of all ages, myself included, invariably caught red handed, or wet headed as the case may be, forced to spend days and nights unbearably burdened with greasy, stringy, untouchable hair.

Despite the impeccable reputation of this expensive, well recommended private girl's school, we were driven by the quite appalling food selections to the drastic measure of lining our uniform jacket pockets with plastic, sneaking the inedible food out to unload the offensive stuff in the bushes at the first opportunity, ideally undetected.

Without a whip or a visible threat, this headmistress ruled by icy stares and clipped voice alone. I will not easily forget the day an Irish classmate and I climbed out the second story bathroom window, then with some difficulty hopped onto the roof of a nearby shed to catch three rays of sunshine; the only time I remember seeing the sun in that entire school year.

During our descent from the shed roof, I leaped off light as a gazelle, landed on the ground and turned just in time to see my friend disappear through the roof in a cloud of black smoke. Rooted to the spot in shock, it took me a moment to realize that she had not chosen this rapid manner of descent… the roof must have given way.

Peering through a blackened window of the shed to see where she had landed and whether she was hurt, I was astounded to see she had fallen a distance of about ten feet, landing on a pile of coal in the locked shed…there she was, barely visible, a black rag doll with spiky red hair, sitting with legs askew under a settling cloud of coal dust.

The face smiled, a row of teeth appeared, and we both doubled up on either side of the window in helpless laughter, more from fear and shock than actual merriment. We still had to get her out, and someone would have to explain the gaping hole in the roof. In for a penny, in for a pound, I broke the window and helped her out.

At lunch assembly the next day, a tight-lipped Headmistress announced that no one would eat until the culprits who put the three-foot hole in the roof of the coal shed announced themselves. There was no way out of it, we confessed, and were invited to an interview in the wood paneled den of the lioness that very afternoon. My terrified friend sat outside the office on a hard wooden bench, bent over with stomach cramps from fear, as I knocked on the massive dark wooden door.

Inside the office of doom I stood as tall as possible, with an air of solemn dignity, until the Headmistress asked what we were doing on the roof. The moment she said the word *roof,* my mind filled with the image… the surprised face and red hair disappearing through the hole in a cloud of black smoke. Bursting into a fit of giggles, convulsing in fact, choking, tears streaming with the effort not to laugh, I fell backwards into a chair where I covered my face with my hands, shaking uncontrollably with muffled laughter. Somehow that mad display saved me.

Stern and unbending, the essence of English 'stiff upper lip', yet still somehow a granny, with her soft skin and beautifully coiffed white hair, it was this elegant Headmistress' job to instill compliance in one hundred or so spirited girls from the ages of eight to seventeen. Usually she accomplished this to perfection using only killing looks and a soft voice that somehow spoke of untold menace. Now she was shocked into silence, speechless. No one had heard laughter in that office for years, the walls were dripping with the echoes of past student's fears.

Our punishment was not expulsion as we expected. A novel chastisement was found for our novel crime. My parents had resolved their differences long enough to find this medieval school, and when father dropped me there and met the Headmistress, they found each other mutually charming. That and the distance he had come to meet her played an important part in her decision not to kick me out.

She deemed it unfair to throw out the Irish girl and not me, so we both found ourselves relegated to sitting outside the Headmistress' office window where she could keep an eye on us, during lunch, recesses and free periods… for weeks, in all kinds of weather, very little of it good.

I can't say the school experience harmed me, getting away from Malibu for a while probably turned out to be a good move, although not one I would have chosen. Peace had been restored when I returned like the Prodigal Daughter. Both parents were amused at my stories and mystified why I didn't complain about the odd rules. What the heck, it was only for a school year, and I'd learned that almost anything could be endured if the end is in sight.

The following summer in Malibu was a relatively peaceful one by all standards, although parental tensions were still abounding. In September I went off to boarding school again, this time to the South of France. *Cours Maintenant* was an international school situated high on a hill above the Croisette in Cannes, and attracted students from far-flung corners of the world; Iran (as it was called then) Saudi Arabia, Italy, Japan and the U.S.

Father had friends in Cannes, and my maternal grandmother was only a few miles up the coast in Monte Carlo, so I did not feel too lost, although rather like a puppy tossed into a pond, it was sink or swim. I had to get the unfamiliar language under control quickly, or remain mute. I learned quite a bit of French in quite a short time, and was soon comfortable chatting on most subjects. When the entire family made the move to France a couple of years later, there was no stopping me, and I am happy to say I still speak French like a native.

My best friends at school in Cannes were two tall blond American girls, sisters, who took me with them on weekends to visit their father on the Flagship of the Sixth Fleet stationed in nearby Villefranche. He was the Captain (or was he perhaps an Admiral? My apologies for the memory lapse) of the enormous aircraft carrier he presided over and lived on. I loved these outings. The Captain's dining room was splendiferous. Whenever we had dinner onboard, I marveled at the exquisite china and silver, and the sumptuous meals that were served as elegantly as in the best French Restaurants. Walking to and fro on the decks were dozens of handsome, smartly uniformed men to ogle us… covertly of course, given the status of the girls' father and our tender years.

Life was grand. I don't remember being lonely or homesick, but perhaps I was, or why else would I be caught shoplifting candy and a lipstick from a store, necessitating a trip to France for father to sort things out? When he asked me why I would do such a thing, my answer puzzled us both. "I didn't want to ask you for money." We both knew the school held funds for me.

It was in Cannes at the age of fifteen or so that I was first introduced to men/men relationships. Not on the aircraft carrier I am quick to point out, but at the beach, the odd stony beaches that make up the coast all along the South of France, beaches where no one actually *sits* on the beach, and lounge chairs are *de rigeur*.

Each portion of the beach is owned by a different concessionaire; thus different restaurants, different colored towels and umbrellas, and different kinds of people make a bright patchwork up and down La Croisette, the famous boardwalk stretching from one end of town to the other.

Sitting on the obligatory lounge chair with a girlfriend one Saturday afternoon, lunch and fruit juice on the table between us, we lolled in the preferential treatment afforded us because her father owned the beach concession.

I remarked that there were some very good looking guys at the beach next door, and so many of them! My girlfriend laughed and said

"Well that's because it's a gay beach."

Not sure of my ground here I said, "What do you mean?" She pointed out two handsome young guys spreading sun tan oil on each other…

"See, they are together, boyfriend and girlfriend." Being yet a virgin, (and remaining so for a few more years) with no personal knowledge of sexual relationships, the whole thing went right over my head, and is as unimportant yet slightly puzzling to me today as it was then.

I returned to Malibu at the end of the school year with prized possessions…the latest in French Bikini's. One was a black and white check pattern with buttons sewn all over it. I don't know if it was the uniqueness of the buttons, or the size of the skimpy bikini that hadn't yet hit Malibu shores, but I soon got a taste of what it is to be the center of things.

Whenever family and friends got together on the beach, I basked in the attention that my new little strips of French fabric brought me, paying no heed at all to the disapproving glares of married women in their suddenly matronly late sixties suits… feeling instead a sense of odd elation when they clipped their husbands on the shin for a roving eye. Suddenly I was sexy, sixteen, and a magnet for teenage trouble.

While the gears were grinding to get us all off to the healthy atmosphere of the French Countryside… castle found, moving vibrations in the air, Bekins boxes in every hallway…I still had time to have one close encounter with disaster. A TV series was being filmed down the road called *77 Sunset Strip*. My friends and I, in that precarious place in time between kids and young adults, spent a few hours watching the filming, and became friendly with some of the cast. One of the assistant producers, a tall nice looking guy in his thirties, asked if I would like to spend the next day on the set with him. I was thrilled to be thus honored, and when he came to the house the next day to meet my parents and asked if I could spend the day watching them film the show, they said that would be fine.

I managed to suppress any awe of my first limo ride, and was only slightly disappointed to notice the Driver was not in attendance; instead my new 'friend' was doing the driving, so we were both in the front seat rather than the cushy 'star department' in back. I had been looking forward to that.

Not paying much attention to where we were going until we turned onto Crosscreek Road, I was slightly surprised to find he knew this private lane, and even more surprised when he parked the limo under a shady tree and led me to the secret little beach on the edge of the stream. The beach Raindaughter had so obligingly deposited for the pleasure of her favorite children. Today there was no one about, no screams of laughter, no chatting or giggling. Just peaceful silence on this sunny pretty day. Puzzled but compliant, I sat on the beach with him as he requested, wondering, still hopeful that the movie crew would show up and my day on the set would materialize as promised. Compared to my one hundred pounds, this man at over six feet tall had no trouble at all quickly wrapping his arms around me and pinning me to the beach beneath him.

There I lay, silent and mystified while this large pleasant man groped and kissed me (my only experience with kissing had been among my peers…why would an older man want to kiss a young kid?) I was not scared at this point, in fact I don't ever remember being scared, only embarrassed… particularly when a large booming voice thundered through the high reeds separating us from the road … "Hello, are you allright?!"

Well, yes I was allright thank you, just madly embarrassed, and who wanted to know?? Extricating myself from the now distracted giant, I hopped up, adjusting my jean shorts which were still intact but stretched where groping hands had tried in vain to make an entrance.

The owner of the booming voice appeared at my side, dressed in the impressive uniform of the Malibu Sheriff Department. He pulled me next to him, and with the most piercing look at the tussled man towering above me, repeated his question to me more quietly… "Are you allright?"

Not quite sure anymore, finally realizing how close I had come to my first brush with danger, real danger, I allowed myself to be led to the police car parked next to the limo. The tears came then, how much in embarrassment at my naiveté, or the fear of my parents finding out, I cannot say.

I begged the police officer, (once again my savior, and me without my horse) not to tell my parents. As there were no further repercussions, apart from the frequent flashes of mortification I had to deal with when the episode relived itself in my memory, I believe he did not tell them.

Suddenly the talk of a move to France became a rushing reality. The Castle had been purchased over the summer, our beautiful Malibu home was on the market, things were moving fast... too fast... yet probably just in time.

With all the kids to keep track of, with all the trips, the horseback riding, the meals prepared and eaten together, I do not remember a single time when my mother sat me down and told me there were a lot of things a teenage girl needed to look out for...I am not saying she didn't do it, I am saying I do not remember it, and would be inclined to believe that is because heart to heart talks, parent to teenager, were not on the agenda in those days.

Certainly nothing in the vein of the numerous "Life Lessons" I foist on my daughter at every opportunity. 'How to be kind, when to be careful, to save her trust for true friends'...at which she grumbles "Oh Mom, not another Life Lesson!" Yet I have proof that she listens.

Compiling a few of these Life Lessons one day, I thought to send them to a few parenting magazine, to share with all the mothers and teenagers who make up their vast audiences. Instead, as the book developed, it seemed to ask for the motherly words of wisdom somewhere about here...and I will be quite content if they are of value to only one person, wherever they are needed...

To My Beautiful Teenage Daughter
Thoughts from Me to You

New friends are pavestones on the adventurous path to who you are…their different viewpoints, ideas, and lifestyles will mingle with yours; **accept the best, leave the rest.**

Romance can be scary, exciting, puzzling and wonderful; it should also be **fun**. If it isn't, step away.

Don't give too much of yourself… emotionally or physically in the beginning of a relationship, ideally, **explore and have fun** without getting hurt, or unduly hurting another.

Don't agonize over blowups, breakups, or misunderstandings; you are young, **learning, watching, and testing.**

Trust another with your **secrets and dreams** only when you are sure it is a **real friendship.**

'Teasing' one another about secrets or faults is ok in **private;** it is a breach of trust to do so in front of others.

Spend time with people who love and care for you, and have your best interests at heart.

In all relationships, whether Family, Friends or Work, be determined to **focus on the good aspects,** let the small negatives slide.

A great friendship/relationship = both parties feel good about themselves, secure in their support of one another… **both bring out the best in one another.**

R E S P E C T is still the key word.

<u>It is wise NOT to spend time with anyone who;</u>

Threatens or pressure you in any way,

Tries to **separate** you from your friends and family,

Dislikes **their own family.** Even if they have good reason, the trouble will be deep rooted and too strong to handle at this time in your life,

Expects you to **solve their problems;** money, family, addictions, etc. If this crops up during marriage, then you must do your best to help; keeping an eye on when to **bail out** if you can not help, or your peace of mind is being destroyed,

Does not **support your goals and dreams,** or who stifles your sense of purpose;

Has a vastly **different cultural background,** whose values or religious beliefs would be difficult to accept or adapt to.

With all my love, MUM

MUNCHKINS & SKY SWINGS

I believe both of my parents thought the move from California to the French countryside would place their children in a more healthy, more natural environment, and perhaps restore the troubled marriage… that a new, oh so different environment might refresh the crackled, dry paste that was barely holding their union together.

I do not think either of them realized the challenges and difficulties laying ahead for my mother, brusquely dropped into the life of a Chatelaine, mistress of a huge unheated castle, smack in the middle of the French countryside. Beautiful yes, but bereft of the amenities so taken for granted in her California lifestyle.

To make matters exceedingly complicated for her, while father was fluent in French…and I had picked up more than a smattering of the language at boarding school, mother didn't speak enough French even to buy bread without being subjected to curious stares from the village shopkeepers. She didn't have a clue where to start looking for beds and furniture… small details father may have forgotten in his enthusiasm to move to France.

Mother wasn't at all sure how long she could, or would, continue cooking for ten or more people every day on a wood-burning stove, even though it was a huge eight burner showpiece, previously the mainstay of an excellent nearby restaurant.

She was miserable, homesick for her familiar California life, and furious at being dependent on Father to get even minor things done. Seeing him so at home in this environment… his Mother was

French and he had grown up speaking the language… did not ease her frustration. I don't remember hearing or seeing them engage in any meaningful conversations about her predicament, although I once saw a kettle of hot water flying across the kitchen in the general direction of Father's head.

The trip from Malibu to France had been an adventure from which Mother was still recovering. Highlights of this expedition flash through my mind at the slightest provocation, and even now, still make me smile. To my mother however, responsible for everyone's safety and comfort, it must have been a project that cried out for Prozac.

Take the vision of my sister's horse dangling in the air from a crane high above the New York docks. Jenny's white horse 'Silver,' and another pretty bay filly had traveled by truck cross-country from Malibu to New York, arriving in time to be loaded onboard a ship for the ocean part of the voyage to Marseille, our first stop on French soil. This 'horse move' must have necessitated days of planning so that parents, kids, dogs, and the extra Malibu neighbor arrived by plane from Los Angeles in time to meet the horse truck at the New York docks. Frankly, I have no idea how my parents orchestrated this feat.

After the human elements of the family arrived at JFK airport, there must have been a day of rest and regrouping, however I only remember us all miraculously gathering at the cruise ship docks in New York, where we watched, rigid with tension, as the horses in individual box stalls were hoisted in midair by a crane, then swung out onto the forward deck of the Zim Lines cruise ship… the only Cruise Company father found that was willing to allow the horses on deck. Under the watchful eyes of the Captain from his lofty bridge, we were able to visit the horses every day, feed them and clean out their boxes, (over the railing… trust fish and marine plants can use a little manure). God bless that kind Captain.

We were underway, out at sea and well into the fourth day of the nine-day cruise. The dogs were tied up on deck outside our cabins, when they escaped; all three of them. The stewards had been happily giving them snacks and playing with them when they suddenly went AWOL.

Thrilled with their escapade, finally able to have a good stretch (our daily ten minute walkabouts obviously counted for nothing), they tore joyfully around the deck, barking their heads off, then plummeted into the swimming pool area at top speed. The Saint Bernard didn't lose a beat. She enthusiastically romped through and over the deck chairs, used and unused, causing several older ladies to clamber up on whatever they could find, screaming for help, *"There's a lion! A lion on the loose, help!"*

An understandable mistake, given the size of the dog and the overall 'bouncyness' of this hundred and fifty pound brute, gentle though she was. Kids, parents and stewards scrambled to catch the escapees…lots of red faces, an embarrassing flap, apologies in order all around, and ironically the dogs suddenly became the much loved celebrities of the ship. Plied with food scraps on the sly by half the passengers now as well as the stewards, it is a wonder they were able to waddle off the ship when we landed in Marseilles.

We were met at the dock by a chartered bus for the family and a truck for the horses to begin the next portion of the journey. We waited on the busy commercial French dock for the horses to be lifted onto solid ground again… the crane and boxstall caper was familiar now, but no less enthralling in reverse. Suddenly Nana, (named I believe for the St. Bernard in Peter Pan, otherwise why such a silly name for a huge dog?) once again managed to get into a great mess.

Tired of the noisy mass of dock workers shouting in a language that made no sense to her, and seeing no apparent progress in the area of getting her family underway and off the docks, Nana spotted a pile of hundred pound burlap sacks of brown sugar, stacked neatly against a warehouse in the shade. She decided to take a nap, and before anyone noticed what she was up to, she had burrowed into the lower sugar bags, ripping one of them wide open. When mother finally noticed her and gave a shriek, Nana was up to her big brown eyes in thick-grained cane sugar, tail thumping happily, once again wondering what all the fuss was about.

Free of the constraints of the cruise ship that brought us from New York to France, horses now safely on terra firma, we happily clambered into the next portion of the expedition, a comfortable bus with great scenic windows. Our entourage included three dogs, seven kids and four adults including David, the extra Malibu bachelor, and Aldo… an intrigued and intriguing Italian passenger from the ship. Aldo joined up with our circus in order to see the adventure to its final destination.

We drove many long hours past French fields of giant sunflowers and lazy cows, through the beautiful sunny towns of Aix en Provence, Nimes, Montpellier and Carcassone, followed closely all the way by a truck carrying the two horses. Descriptions of pit stops for food and other necessities with this menagerie will be left to your imagination, as nothing I can say will completely convey the chaos.

Onwards through the city of Toulouse, then deeper into the French countryside we went…Montauban, Cahors, and right on through the heart of France to the spectacular Medieval town of Sarlat, where my two little brothers, when they were older, would be enrolled in the school run by Jesuit priests.

The last real town our caravan rolled through was Les Eyzies, famous for its prehistoric cave dwellings, probably home to friends of the huge stone Cro Magnon Man, lumbering upright at the foot of the mountain bordering the town …the same stone giant that looks longingly out across the river for his kin. He is also known as the Mousterian Man, and a few miles further we arrived at le Moustier, the last little village of this journey, our Great Trek.

Turning hard right onto a twisting little lane behind a fragrant bakery, we headed carefully up a winding road for a mile or so, to a plateau at the top of a mountain. The bus continued on for a few minutes while we quietly admired the valley views below on either side. There had been no other cars on this narrow little road since we left the patchwork valley below, so we were surprised when the procession suddenly stopped. After hours of driving, the bus and horse truck just stopped in the middle of nowhere.

Upon closer inspection, there appeared to be a driveway camouflaged by enormous trees on either side. Trees that looked like the giant Sequoias we knew from California. These turned out in fact to be a close relation, some of them so old they had been protecting this entrance to a hidden Castle for over a hundred years.

No more tarmac now, but a sandy colored limestone road that seemed part of nature, shaded by an arch of towering Cedars flanking either side of the lane as far as the eye could see. Father asked us all to get out of the bus. Finally so close, he wants to savor our discovery of his dream; and what better way than to abandon the vehicles and *walk* this majestic shaded driveway together.

And so it was, following the yellow sand road not unlike the one in the Wizard of Oz, skipping hand in hand through the sunlight flitting down through tall ferns and Chestnut trees, the seven Benson Munchkins traveled this path together for the very first time. Alternating between moments of awed silence and enthusiastic screams of delight, we walked, skipped and ran the length of the sun dappled driveway. Suddenly, very unexpectedly, we came upon a great stone wall looming fifteen feet high in front of us; huge squares of golden stone divided by massive wooden studded doors ten feet high and twelve feet across. Welcome to the courtyard gates of Chateau de Chaban!

Hanging from a tall tree outside the gates was a swing, a castle size swing. Thick ropes headed for the sky, disappearing amidst the leafy canopy, finally anchoring thirty feet above the ground to a limb the width of a man. Only Superman or a Mad English Scientist could have engineered the realization of such a fantasy just to please his children.

We are thrilled, we are enchanted, *we are through the gates*!

The courtyard and Castle are out of a movie… lavender Wisteria vines outline stained glass windows, turrets and towers tease the skyline, a medieval well waits patiently for us to discover its murky depths, and tucked away in a corner under flowering vines I was not familiar with was a little stone cottage that now magically housed all our riding gear, saddles, bridles, currycombs, the lot.

Father is jumping up and down with excitement…how many times in your life are you truly able to realize your dreams? Father's dream became a reality the moment he saw us fall in love with his Castle.

"Go and pick a room," he shouted, and *en masse* we dashed through the wide stone entrance. The pushing and shoving to be the first inside was viewed with amusement by the silent stone stairway; large wide steps worn down an inch or two in the center from centuries of stomping feet… steps that are glad to be useful again.

There was no squabbling about which room went to whom, they were all magnificent. Jenny and I chose the big square southern tower, me on the first floor, she right above me on the second.

Our matching French windows, eight feet high, opened onto a vista I will always be able to see in my mind's eye…rolling pastures, spectacular trees, a little stream at the base of the valley, and up the other mountainside to another castle, not sitting high and proud like Chaban, but nestled into the forests halfway to the top.

My brother Peter chose the third floor, never taking into consideration the huge flight of shining dark wood stairs on this side of the Castle, stairs he would have to run up and down dozens of times a day. The two little boys, Kit and Keith, chose the room next to Peter's. They were like two peas in a pod and happiest when together.

Wendy and Heather Anne found rooms to their liking in another wing altogether. Father and Mother had splendid chambers on the top floor of yet a third wing, their bedroom alone the size of a normal house. The extra bachelor, David Brown, claimed a beautiful room two floors below with its own entrance and sitting rooms. Two large rooms still remained for guests, which was lucky as the spare Italian, Also, spent a month or so with us before returning to Italy to resume his own life.

This was June in France, and in the first relatively happy months, the joy of these wide open spaces, the unlimited places of discovery and delight, lulled everyone into a state of blissful peace..

Suddenly the weather became 'brisk' to use an understated British term, then it became downright cold, something none of us knew much about, nor apparently were ready for. I took off for Italy.

Rome sounded a lot warmer than France - sunny Italy and all that, or was it the chill in the atmosphere at Chaban that caused me to want to flee? Gemini's are good at fleeing, any excuse at all will do. I asked Father to find me a job there through his friend at the Olivetti Company. Before I had time to change my mind, I found myself in Rome, working for a company near Trastevere that manufactured aeronautical optical equipment.

The company had an important customer base in the U.S. so I wrote or proofread English correspondence for them, did odd office jobs as needed, and proved an asset by spotting a typo on their Italian letterhead that had gone unnoticed for years… it proclaimed they had an office in the *"Untied"* States of America.

The lovely old Italian gentleman from Olivetti was not sure what to do with the responsibility of a California teenager, and recommended I be put in 'safe' lodgings for the first few months. This turned out to be a small convent in the heart of Rome where the nuns took in boarders, girls only. Winter weather was no better here than in France as I soon found out. It is bitter cold *everywhere in Europe in the winter!* But I was far from the pending catastrophe at the Castle, and that suited me fine.

The convent I was housed in for safekeeping was something out of a Dickens novel. It was located deep in the old part of the Roman city, and run by nuns… and there any semblance of a nunnery ended.

The girls stole from one another on a daily basis, the only way to keep things safe was to keep a bag on your person at all times, even when sleeping. There was no discernable heating. The bathroom had long steel horse-trough affairs to wash in, cold water only. The mattresses were made of some kind of burlap, stuffed with horsehair… yes, horsehair. The sheets were of cotton so rough it was like slipping between two blocks of sandy ice, and blankets were something to be fought over. The California life was looking better every day.

As most of the girls had jobs, we were free to come and go in the daytime. Anyone not inside the huge gates by 11:00pm would be locked out for the night.

Needless to say, in pretty quick order one of the other girls and I joined forces and found an apartment to share not far from work. It had heaters and hot water, and life became more normal.

Walking home from work each day I passed a bakery that specialized in pizza. Pizza in Italy then was nothing like pizza in England or the U.S. This was baked in a square pan, with no toppings at all. It was pulled out of the stone oven piping hot, cut into 4x6 inch pieces, sprinkled with olive oil, salt, and upon request, olives… *basta!* That was it.

The taste was too excellent to be put into words. Suffice to say that walking home from the office, I bought an entire kilo at least three times a week. By my math that is a little over two pounds of pizza, and I ate every bite… and still remember the flavor as I write. It is a wonder my figure never moved from its curvy 110 lbs., perhaps the walking balanced things out.

I met my fiancé, Roberto, within the first few months of life in Rome. I had learned enough of the language not to embarrass myself, enough to be able to converse fairly adequately with this interesting Italian. Angular faced, strongly opinionated, and handsome as only Italians can be, he taught me to drive his fivespeed, red Alfa Romeo, and shoot a pistol with great accuracy, although not on the same day. He also improved my fluency in Italian by 100%. I definitely recommend having an Italian fiancé over language courses anytime.

Roberto had inherited a beautiful two-story house from his parents when they died in a car accident several years before we met. He was twenty five and seemingly at peace with the absence of his parents. The aunt that looked after him as a teenager was relieved to find he was happy with me and no longer living alone, and I was oh so glad to be pulled out of the bachelorette life, and into his cozy home.

I am puzzled to find that while I remember perfectly the exquisite taste of that pizza, I cannot remember whether the house was located in Trastevere, or Parioli; both beautiful areas that come to mind one as quickly as the other, so it is not of great importance.

Roberto accompanied me on several visits to Chaban. He drove the Alfa from Rome to Paris, then courageously let me drive the next seven hours, wending down from Orleans through Chateauroux and into Limoges, where we would make a stop to add a dish or place setting to my collection of Limoges Haviland china. The pattern is *Golden Quail*, intricate little gold and lavender spotted quail cavorting among aqua flowers on stunning scalloped platters and plates. While researching the pattern recently I came across replacement prices, and was stunned to see how much each plate is worth now. Beautiful china that I would like my daughter to use and love some day as much as I do.

There were very few 'Autoroutes' at the time. Most of the drive was along those beautiful but dangerous three-lane roads, where French drivers take turns at the national sport of Chicken. Roberto kept his cool while I learned to overtake slower vehicles, which meant anything going less than 90mph. Vehicles from the opposite direction were using the same center passing lane for the same purpose, which made the process very lively.

Judging speed, distance and timing with an expert eye, the winner of the game was the last car to glide in front of the vehicles in his lane, usually fractions of a second before the oncoming car sped by. This was accomplished successfully by all for the most part…the misses were invariably fatal.

From Limoges it was another hour to the Castle along roads twisting through shady chestnut forests. I thought Roberto was extremely brave to let me have the wheel of his precious car, teaching me to navigate the five speed gears and deal with both French and Italian drivers, although some might say they are one and the same.

My family thought Roberto was the cat's meeow. My handsome Italian fiancé and I slept in separate rooms in the Castle to uphold whatever vestige of morals my siblings might have grasped despite the soap opera quality of their young lives. By day we walked in the crisp winter forests, breathing fumes like ice dragons. Our strolls took us through the crystallized vineyards and into the lovely stone barn where enormous wooden vats black with age and the juice of millions of grapes waited patiently for the next Vendange.

Back in the castle, we explored the hidden 'Oubliette', roughly translated as The Forgettery. The wine cellar was large, damp, and dark, a room of stone with an intoxicating and irresistible smell wafting from the rows of bottles and kegs stashed in varying degrees of perfection. When the heavy wooden door was open to the cellar, cleverly hidden behind it was a short, low tunnel that ended suddenly and without any warning at a twenty foot drop into the darkest pit imaginable. The 'oubliette' was where medieval hosts were said to stash unwanted guests. We did in fact find bones in the pit while doing some exploratory digging with shovels, flashlights and buckets, but never determined of what variety.

Roberto and I rode horseback every day in the afternoon when it was warm. Within a month or two of moving to France, my parents had acquired several horses, putting them into the pasture to frolic with the two we brought from California. A large strapping bay for my father, ponies for the smaller kids, and three beauties saved from the butcher's killing fields.

No one asks what kind of horse they are eating in French restaurants; butchers buy 'on the hoof' and by the pound, often ending up with handsome young horses sold to them for reasons one can not imagine. So we saved as many as we could. These new additions to the family got along well with our original imports, Silver, my sister Jenny's quarter-horse, and the beautiful young bay filly we planned to use for breeding.

They made a happy little herd, and what a life they had… munching their way from pasture to pasture in the summer, a dip in the stream for cool fresh water, a bit of exercise on hair-raising gallops through the forests on family rides, slipping and sliding like kids when they awakened one day to find snow on the ground… horse life was good.

So it was a surprise when Father's bay tried to commit suicide one day. He was waiting to be saddled up, tied sloppily to a tree, no doubt without the correct 'easy pull' knot we were taught to use, when some figment of his horsy imagination saw *a scary thing*. He sat back on his haunches and tried to break the rope around his neck… understanding nothing of the laws of ropes and necks.

The noose tightened and his eyes began to bulge; a good smack on the backside to move him forward had absolutely no effect, this was a big horse. I found myself moving as if in a dream…in a daze of shock, watching, seeing, knowing what was happening yet powerless to help. The lightning moves of Roberto saved the Bay that day.

Sensing in a flash the frantic horse could not be wrestled, pulled or pushed forward, he raced to the kitchen a good fifty yards away, grabbed a knife and was back in time to hack the taut, singing rope in half; sending a ton of straining horseflesh crashing backwards to the ground.

The world began to move and spin again. We clawed the rope off the bay's neck while he was still on the ground, jumping back as he staggered up… slowly, a mere semblance of his former majestic self. He stood still as stone for ten seconds, then shook himself as if to get rid of a bad dream, then off he went, cantering around the pasture with his tail held high… quite proud of himself for reasons that we could not fathom..

Back in Italy, Roberto and I split up sometime thereafter, although I can't remember exactly why I let that happen as he was a remarkably great guy. I remember he wanted to move to California and learn the computer business from someone my father introduced him to, and I wanted to stay in Europe. Or perhaps more honestly, I did not want to be with him while he took the baby steps needed before he would be as cool in California as he was in Italy and France. I knew he would have to learn English, find a place to live, cope with a new job, all things most women would expect to do when starting out together with their partner. Was I really that selfish?! I can hardly stand to remember being so cavalier with his life, and of course my own. Maybe, just maybe, I simply could not face being uprooted again.

Whatever the reasons, I kissed him goodbye, told him to "Let me know when you get settled there," and said I would join him. And that was the last he saw of me.

I returned to France and sent our engagement ring back to him in California via a friend, a really beautiful ring that belonged to his mother; antique sapphires and diamonds set in platinum. Heartless I may appear, fickle I may be…unfair I am not. He asked me to join him, I chose not to; it never crossed my mind to keep the ring.

A BREAST WORTH 250 FRANCS

I found a nice apartment in Paris and got a job with a U.S. Law firm specializing in American movies being made in Europe. I visited Chaban often, driving south one or two weekends a month in the red Alfa. My red Alfa now. Before Roberto left for California, father bought if for me at a 'family price'. The last time Roberto and I were at Chaban together, the Alfa had been parked in the courtyard entrance for the night. Someone climbed up the huge pile of logs stocked for firewood on either side of the entrance, and accidentally toppled a large log onto the Alfa's classic front right fender, creating a very unclassic dent. A French *artiste* restored the fender perfectly to my eyes, and Roberto left happily for California knowing his baby was in good hands.

Mastering the skill of driving in Paris without Roberto's calming voice was a real challenge. The *piece de resistance* had to be without a doubt circling around the Arc de Triomphe's seven lanes in one piece. One of Paris' best loved architectural marvels, the Arc is also an irresistible target for daredevil flyboys in small planes, illegally winging through the high arch with only a few feet to spare.

Napoleon Bonaparte started construction of the monument in 1806 to honor his own military victories and soldiers in the French Revolutionary. Work faltered as his troops began to suffer defeats, and it was not completed until 1836 under the reign of King Louis Philippe. Napoleon never did march triumphantly through the monument as planned; only his remains passed under the Arch in December 1840 on the way to his final resting place at *Les Invalides.*

Since then famous victory marches around or under the Arc included the French and Allies in 1944 and 1945. A United States postage stamp of 1945 shows the *Arc de Triomphe in the background as victorious American troops march down the Champs-Élysées and U.S. airplanes fly overhead on 29 August 1944.*

From the rooftop view of this military monument, Paris is spread out in all its glorious 360 degrees. Radiating out from the monument, North, South, East, and West, are many - way too many, busy streets, twelve to be exact. The largest by far is the immensely wide Champs Elysees, whose numerous lanes march triumphantly from the center of the Arc, straight as a yardstick for a mile and a half, ending in a wide circle around the fountain of Place de La Concorde.

The Arc is also affectionately known as *L'Etoile,* the Star, with its twelve Avenues reaching out from the center. The most well known after the Champs Elysees is probably Avenue Foch, in honor of the Commander in Chief of the Allied Armies in France who accepted the German surrender in World War I.

Avenue Victor Hugo is next, named after France's most celebrated romance writer and poet of his era… Kleber, Icna, Marceau, a dizzying array of famous French names flash by at tremendous speed when seen from a car negotiating its perilous lanes. Converging from all over Paris at the perimeter of the Etoile, the avenues spew hundreds of cars into the melee circling around the monument in a speeding mass of unrelenting vehicles. Those in the know deftly maneuver from one lane to another in time to spin off at the desired exit, the less bold just keep on spinning and praying…the French version of the Mad Hatter teacup ride.

There are stories of tourists in rental cars being stuck in this great circle for hours, going round and around, too timid to blast their way across the incoming lanes of traffic to get off at any street, let alone the one they were aiming for. I am proud to say I have only ever made one unnecessary panic circle around the Arc de Triomphe.

I admit I was lucky. The first time I drove the Alfa in Paris without Roberto was in August, a blissfully quiet time when all the Parisians head for the South of France. (All it would seem, to the same places…Nice, Cannes, Cap D'antibes, Beauleu, St. Tropez, you can not walk anywhere along the French Riviera in the summertime without tripping over Parisians).

Getting around the Etoile was a breeze in August… there were so few cars that my confidence soared as the famous street names spun by in their intricate circle, and my street of choice was deftly darted into without a single close encounter. By the time the Parisians flocked back to their roost, I had mastered L'Etoile, it was now my monument. All other cars were intruders to be handled with the calm, detached air that belies any possible bluffing.

Summertime in Europe takes on an entire lifestyle of its own. Whether in a villa in the countryside or at the coastal resorts, no one counts the hours, nor notices whether one is waking or sleeping. The skies do not get dark til after ten pm, the mornings are for crisp walks and nature appreciation, for breakfast at small cafés, with their delectable buttery croissants…dipped, depending on your country of origin, in blistering hot coffee or sweet hot chocolate. Or you could sleep til noon, and rise just in time for a swim and a long lunch, another favorite pastime on a lazy summer day.

There are too many beautiful towns to explore along the European coasts, each one prettier than the last. The romantic names were but a day's drive from the castle in my speedy little Alfa. Sometimes alone, but more often with a girlfriend from Paris, I would head off through Provence and Montpellier, past the marshy salt flats of Camarque with their famous wild horses, and finally to the ritzy little seaside towns… Nice, Cannes, Antibes, Beauliu, St. Jean Cap Ferrat, Villefranch and St Tropez.

Although most of the beaches along the coast are considered bathing suit tops 'optional', there was an archaic law, still in effect in my day, that topless was not allowed. Tahiti Beach in St. Tropez, one of the most well known for its topless ladies, was therefore the most likely to be subjected to the occasional raid by the French police, undoubtedly for them a pleasant change from the tedious whistle blowing and arm waving for which they are so well known. I feel grateful to have actually been on Tahiti Beach one day when two fully dressed *Gendarmes* come stomping along the shoreline in full uniform and polished black shoes… a completely ridiculous sight that nonetheless sent all topless ladies scurrying for a wrap to cover their breasts. The fine was 250 francs **per exposed breast**… in the event one could not cover them both in time. This worked out to about $50 each, and I defy any man to find a single breast at a better price.

Sitting ten feet away from me on the beach was Mme de R… a lovely young lady married to a man whose name is well known on all continents. Caught offguard, she was fined just that amount; 250 francs for one perfect breast jutting out through the folds of a casually draped diaphanous wrap… the perky nipple refusing to bow to the indignity of such a rushed cover up. Her 250 franc fine was the subject of much amusement over beachside lunches of grilled crayfish and crisp, multi-leafed salads.

Continuing along the coast to Monte Carlo, I always spent a few days with my mother's parents, a spot of high luxury in our otherwise modest choice of accommodations along the way; humble but homey little hotels, made more than acceptable with their delicious *petits dejeuners* of croissants and choice of hot beverage.

I would be fibbing if I said we *always* traveled modestly, often we met up with friends on yachts, and sailed the Mediterranean on acres of teak and blood red sails. Gianni Agnelli, the original owner of the Fiat car company had such a yacht, forgive me if I have lost the name, but the thrill of the wind in *those* sails is still with me.

And the nightclubs along the Riviera… there was nothing modest about them, from any viewpoint. Barely-there outfits, perfect tans and perfect bodies, the men as beautiful as the women. I met the *sexiest* young Italian playboy in our favorite hot spot in St. Tropez one night. My girlfriend and I hopped into his Maserati and screamed over the tiny lanes to his rented villa. We shed most of our clothes and dived into the Olympic size pool. (Alas, I have never been able to drop the undies for these nocturnal romps, some misplaced vestige of modesty, but there you are.)

When our Italian Stallion could not find the switch to turn off the pool lights, he asked us to walk back up to the villa with him, all of us still *senza vestiti*. After checking around the terrace and exhausting all the usual places the pool light switches might have been installed, he went into one of the many second story bedrooms and came out with a pistol. Walking out on the terrace, he took aim, and casually shot out all the lights in the pool.

"That's better," he said, "*molto megliore,* now let's go swim."

I am not an electrician, but the idea of broken bulbs and underwater sockets did nothing to entice me back into that pool, although I did accompany them to retrieve my clothing. My girlfriend did not seem the least bit intimidated by this turn of events and said she would stay.

It did not even occur to me to ask this lunatic for a ride back to town, I just tossed on my skimpy dress and scampered off down the road, in the pitch dark, shoes in hand, not sure whether to hope for a ride or be ready to jump into a ditch and hide if anyone drove by.

For this was not my first encounter with mad Italians and guns, and I do not refer here to Roberto, who was a completely different animal, and a responsible, kind, considerate person. No, my other gun episode took place in Rome before I met Roberto, and involved a silver-gray convertible Lancia, and the son of one of Italy's well-known vintners.

Frascati? Manchatti?, Patachi?, who can remember the name of the vineyard… I went out to dinner several times with Giancarlo and he was always the perfect gentleman. Teasing me about words I tripped over in Italian, enchanting me with tales of his family's struggles and ultimate success with the vineyard, and whispered confessions of his love for me.

One night he didn't take me straight home as usual. With the top down and the stars above, I wasn't paying much attention to where we were going, I was comfy and happy and thought I knew this man/boy quite well. We came to the top of a hill and a long, lonely lane stretched out ahead of us in the dim light of the half moon. He pulled off the road and stopped, switching off the headlights. He didn't leave me much time to wonder why, just gathered me up in his strong arms for a smooch. Well that was allright, I'd had better and I'd had worse… but I didn't like the way his arms were tightening around me, crushing me, suffocating me.

Smacking him in the chest I pushed out of his grip and came up for air. "What are you doing?" I gasped, "You are choking me."

"I want you" he said, "ti voglio… ti voglio tanto."

"Well you can't force me like that!" I huffed, and without a word, he leaned across to the glove compartment in front of me, opened it and pulled out a pistol, which he pointed it at my head. Before he had finished saying, "I think I can," (credo che si!) I was somehow out over the top of the door, and running; not scampering this time, really running for my life down a narrow Italian lane in the dark, no time for déjà vu. I ducked into a bush to take off my shoes, barefoot Malibu instincts coming to the fore, crouched down and listened. I heard nothing, but could see headlights coming slowly towards me.

Just the lights, moving slowly closer. No noise, the engine only the softest purr. No one calling out, coaxing me, apologizing. Just the light creeping closer. This was not a good sign. Any thoughts I may have had of telling him what an idiot he was and that he could take me home now, vanished.

Ignoring the jabbing sticks in my backside, I kept my eye on the advancing light and snuggled further back into the bushes. The headlights were almost even with me now, the car an invisible sleek dark shape behind the glare. I couldn't stand watching, waiting any longer. I shut my eyes and held my breath, willing my heart not to beat so loudly.

The car rolled on silently by, the crunch of stones against tires betraying its presence. I didn't move a muscle, 'eyes wide shut', and didn't even think to pray. I don't know how long it was before I opened my eyes, then moved an arm, a cramped leg. I must have been in a trance, as the ghostly car had long floated out of sight.

Shaken, and aware of the night noises now, I headed slowly back in the direction we had come.

The lane finally intersected with a well-traveled road, and I again risked my life flagging down a ride. Luck was back in my corner and a very elegant lady drove me to my apartment, after expressing relief that it was not her daughter in my predicament.

A month or so later my father called to say a large case of Italian wine had been delivered to the castle with a note saying, "with my best wishes that you and your family enjoy my small gift."

"Darling" father said, "You have such nice friends!"

Sorry about that little distraction, I seem to have absolutely no control over when these vignettes pop up. I have never told anyone about that near death experience, certainly not my parents at the time. It happened a hundred years ago, I have not talked about it since, so why does it pop up when I am trying to write about a nice scenic drive along the Riviera?

Where were we… oh yes, after Monte Carlo, crossing the small Italian border town of Ventimiglia. Sometimes you can zip through here quite quickly… or not, if it happens to be August, when the lines of cars waiting to pass through customs are backed up for several miles and several hours. With holiday resignation, drivers get out of their cars and use the extra time to initiate a chat with an attractive fellow detainee, so the time is not really wasted after all.

La Spetzia is a tiny jewel nestled in a cliffside curve of the coastal road between Genoa and Roma. My very favorite Italian town is the dreamy hillside village of Positano, lying somewhere along the Amalfi coast, hidden geographically from me for now, as I can't remember how to get there. I do know however, that I spent hours meandering up and down the steep tiny streets devoted entirely to little shops. A cotton fabric with a design unique to the village is made into bags and purses found nowhere else in the world. Outdoor cafes big enough for only three small round tables, tiny bakeries filled with crusty rolls and golden breads, discovered by following ones nose to the unforgettable aroma. I am at this moment unable to locate Positano on the World Atlas, however you probably know where it is.

Or is this quaint, sunny little town spilling down an Italian hillside a figment of my imagination? A fantasy? I think not, and may have to go back there some day to prove it to myself.

SAILING SHIPS AND GREEK ISLES

Having survived a year in Italy, if only barely, I decided to return to The City of Light for a while. I thrived in the more serious, work-oriented atmosphere of Paris. During weekend trips to Chaban I could see that my poor mother was not finding chateau life what it was cut out to be, or at least not at all as it had been portrayed to her by father.

When it became too much to bear, she chose a diversion, or perhaps a consolation, an English boyfriend. Learning nothing from my youthful admonitions in California to be more discreet, she took off with this gentleman (?) for a weekend in London.

It took father about an hour to obtain a court order from the obliging Mayor of the nearest village. Father was an important person in this corner of France; he was revitalizing the area by restoring the ancient stone buildings, employing heretofore out of work villagers as housekeepers and farmhands, and was generally considered an asset worth keeping happy.

The document swiftly put together by the Mayor ordered that our mother was not allowed on the property of Chateau de Chaban, not ever, not to see her children, not even to pick up her clothes. With me away in Paris, Jenny, at the tender age of fourteen, stepped into the Mother Role.

A very miserable year for all, particularly Father. Lonely and angry, he sobbed in his soup that, "He hated all women, he never wanted to see another woman again, we children were his life, he would always be there for us."

A few weeks, after Mum's departure, I drove to Chaban for the weekend, it was now becoming more of a duty than fun. I thought the older kids seemed to be coping, but the little ones could not mask their quiet sadness. Facing me that weekend was the most devastating task in my young life…telling my two littlest brothers, probably five and six at the time, that their mother was not coming home… not now, not soon, not ever.

It had never been mentioned, never properly explained… the children had been holding their breath, waiting for a sign that never came. As days turned into weeks, they hoped against hope Mum would miraculously appear in the courtyard, in the kitchen, on the patio, anywhere… where was she? Was she ever coming back? Everyone hotfooting silently around the subject so as not to give the dreadful thoughts the weight of words.

Engraved in my memory forever, and the source of such sorrow that a vow not to have children of my own was born that day, was the scene in the large oak paneled library… two little blond cherubs sitting in a huge dark red velvet couch, lost in the plump cushions, leaning against one another for support, until the littlest one got up the courage to whisper those dreaded words to me. "When is mummy coming home?"

My voice choked, no words would come out at all… little angels watching intently as I went over and sat next to them, tears not staying out of sight as they should. I struggled to get out some words of comfort, anything that would make it easier for them. Nothing happened, I was mute. Then the wise older brother, all of six, said to his little sidekick "shhh, you're upsetting her." I don't remember any more than that, I pray that I hugged them and cried with them, but I don't remember. That part of my brain is broken forever.

My darling little Kit and Kat, as I still refer to them at our family get-togethers even though they are now strapping men. Why should children ever be put through such agony? How could I not learn from that and see a similar scene looming in my little daughter's future, my vow not to have children luckily broken by love for my husband. I can not forgive myself for repeating my parents' mistakes… when I knew, I KNEW the pain caused all around.

This memory will now be locked away on the dark bottom shelf of my mind's golden gembox.

My pretty girl has not come home yet, and night is falling in Hopetown. It is time to face the fact that I have screwed up. I have a painful divorce to fit in here somewhere (later, later) and the guilt of having thrown away a perfectly good husband pretty much by mistake, leaving me overindulgent in the area of disciplining my only daughter.

Making up for the lack of a father by being extra under-standing, allowing certain rudeness and unfinished chores to go 'unnoticed', I have set myself up for frequent bouts of disrespect. How often have I said to Genevieve "Life is short, let's not waste it in useless arguments, let's have fun together." Yet whenever she went overboard (even by my easy standards), when that adrenaline started rushing in response to her over-the-top rudeness, I admit to having enjoyed - in the past - a surge of angry energy. Enjoyed the power of bending her to my will by my voice alone, brittle and hard enough to crack the heart of a grown man.

In truth it may not have been the voice alone that silenced her retorts and made her draw back in respect, still seething with anger. It could have been "the look" before The Pounce. I am not proud to say that on two occasions in Nassau, I literally pounced on her... pummeled her with my fists; notwithstanding that at five feet eight inches, she is four inches taller than me. I still maintain this was necessary at those moments to break the unforgiving tension between us. She was gracious enough not to fight back, an act that would have led who knows where, given the very short fuse that was my lot at the time, and her far superior strength.

Now I no longer enjoy that power. I have resolved to find a better way to move along in life together, to assure that if one of us were to die unexpectedly, the other would not have to bear the inconsolable grief of Regrets... it is more than enough to live with the infinite pain of Missing.

I ask God's help, and trust that my subconscious will churn out its hidden knowledge, guiding me to achieve this new peaceful goal of living 'strife free' throughout the seasons, with this wondrously tall, golden haired, dimple cheeked fourteen year old to whom I gave life, and who in turn is my life.

Things had gone south at the Castle...Mum was banished, the kids were miserable, and demons were plaguing father. He was sadder than he could ever have imagined about the breakup of his marriage, devastated at being alone to cope with seven children, but determined to stick by his decision.

Although this was long before Hollywood celebrities discovered the charms of Tibet's exiled lamas living precariously in parts of India and Nepal, Father decided to go off on a pilgrimage to the top of the world, to Darjeeling, on the advice of a French business friend, to see a certain Tibetan Buddhist lama.

Father sat in the mountaintop monastery, crosslegged on the floor in front of the very wise, gently smiling Kangjur Rinpoche whom I would later meet. With no translator and no common language, a strong and unequivocal mystical bond was forged between the two men... one shattered and broken, one whole and wise.

I consider myself pretty much out of the picture at home at this point, having been away the year in Italy learning that beautiful language, and now living in Paris... leaving my sister Jenny to deal with the younger children's school, clothes, food and much emotional comfort. I do not remember being any help at all, and in fact unwittingly instigated the next chapter in our complicated lives.

Father returned from India with renewed energy and purpose. He came to Paris to see me, and on a perfectly normal busy Paris day, he met my very charming, very pretty, very busty, red-headed French roommate. He promptly fell in love.

Beautiful Maritee and I had moved into a roomy apartment together a few months after she began working at the same American law firm as I. She was at the end of a going nowhere relationship with a young Frenchman when father turned his vigorous, energetic and enthusiastic attention on her.

Reticent at first to date him, she was perhaps still thinking of her French love, or the difference in age between herself and the father of her roommate. She quickly succumbed however to the obvious advantages of this charming, attentive and irresistible man with a castle, lots of money, and an impressive fleet of vintage cars. Two 1960 Rolls Royce limos, one burgundy, one blue. The electric sliding glass window between the driver's seat and the passengers in the back turned and the out to be a big bonus, shutting out the noise of a carload of unruly kids whenever necessary.

There was a richly upholstered Napier, a sleek black convertible Bentley, another touring Talbot like the one in Malibu, and a zippy Morgan, dark racing green. At least one of these treasures later became part of Prince Rainier's famous collection in Monte Carlo.

Thus in spite of Father's sodden promises after mother's departure that, "You kids are my life and I will always be there for you"… all of a sudden, he wasn't. Now he was in Paris more than at Chaban, and it was a case of "I love you kids a lot, but I'm very busy now, can't you see?"

Father courted Maritee in his irrepressible, enthusiastic way. He was an incurable romantic who wouldn't take no for an answer. I was reminded of the times when Mother was the beneficiary of his love of surprises and generosity in younger, lighter days in Malibu.

One birthday morning he drove with her around the Malibu hills and canyons for half an hour or so before a speck of something shiny on a distant hilltop caught her eye. As they drove closer to have a look, Mother stood up in the convertible to see better, and almost fell out of the car in shock.

Sitting at the crest of a mountaintop, in the middle of nowhere, was a shining blue sports car with a huge red ribbon around it… Triumph's most recent convertible model and Mother's birthday present. How could you not love a man like that?

Now it was Maritee's turn, and Father did not disappoint. Maritee and I were working in a beautiful building, Number One, Place de la Concorde, right around the corner from the famous Restaurant,

Maxim's. Our boss spent many long and productive business lunches there, his success rate proof that it is more effective to negotiate over a perfect Bordeaux wine and exquisite steak *au poivre*, rather than a pedestrian cheeseburger and Coke.

The Concierge of the building telephoned me up in the office one day to say there was a movie being made outside the building, and would Maritee and I please come downstairs. Mystified but curious, we walked through the huge glass doors on the ground floor, and out into a milling crowd, where a movie camera was thrust in our faces. A large black horsedrawn carriage stood waiting at the curb, complete with uniformed coachman.

A bewigged and liveried footman suddenly appeared at our side, presenting Maritee with a deep red velvet cushion trimmed with gold tassels. Nestled on the cushion was a single red rose, and a gold Cartier lighter.

Forever thanking the Gods that her first instinct was to pick up the rose, (as all was being recorded on film, and it would have been unseemingly to "go for the gold" in this case), Mariteee held the rose to her lips and blushed beautifully.

Father swept out of the carriage in a black top hat and cape, and an enormously silly grin on his face. Taking her gently by the arm, he settled her in the carriage and climbed in next to her. The footman jumped on the back of the carriage and held on precariously just like in the movies. The driver cracked a long whip, and the whole entourage took off like the fairy tale it was for a leisurely ride up the Champs Elysees. For a second date, that is hard to beat. The lighter was to replace one Maritee lost on their first date.

Now I knew Father was impossible to say no to, and I was thrilled that he was taking an interest in life again, but nonetheless very concerned that it was too soon for the kids to have to deal with another relationship in their lives. Father and Maritee spent a week at La Reserve Hotel in the South of France, where he apparently climbed from his third story balcony to hers, whether in fun or proof of his love I know not, and risked his life doing so… I thought it was time to speak.

"Father," I said in my most conciliatory, grown up manner, "I am so glad you are happy, just please promise me you will visit Maritee in Paris, and not bring her to Chaban, I just don't think the kids can handle it yet."

"I see your point," he said, "I'll think about it."

Maritee resigned from her job soon thereafter and got her own apartment, and continued to 'date' my father. An actor friend, Roland, moved in with me; an arrangement I thought was perfect… he was incredibly kind, funny, goodlooking, and six feet tall, my favorite height for men.

There was just this tiny, niggly feeling I had that we should be living in *his* apartment…not mine. But he didn't have one. He had been living with family and friends for several months. My inner voice, to whom I paid little heed in those days, was letting me know that aspiring movie directors, whiling away time doing small acting jobs, are not high on the list of future moneymakers, relatively few of them actually achieve their goals, in France at any rate.

Still, he was very handsome, gentle and loving, and my siblings thought he was a hero. Having no brothers or sisters, he treated mine like his own, and got a kick out of being part of our family. So I was willing to wait and see for a bit… a bit turning into a couple of years.

Roland and I met at a café beside a lake just outside of Paris one weekend, several months before I introduced Maritee to father. She and I were having a bite to eat and enjoying the summer sun, when this just stunning guy with the warmest smile asked if he could sit down with us. Apart from a stifled "wow" under my breath, I didn't pay much attention to him, by now quite used to men falling over us to get a peek at Maritees considerable assets. However it gradually became apparent he was actually interested in talking to ME. Maritee was quietly furious, wondering why her boobs hadn't worked their magic, and I was beside myself with glee.

I can't say now if I ever loved Roland, I probably was crazy about him in the beginning, that big goofy grin with the warm soft green eyes and movie star jawline was a killer combination. I definitely wanted him to stick around, he made me look so good. Until his greatest quality became his greatest flaw…he was so easy going that a glass of wine, a piece of cheese and me was all it took to make him happy. That is a lovely take on life, but not a guarantee for success.

I like the beginning better, where everything was going smoothly. I had this hunk of a boyfriend, and although the word had not come into popular use then, he certainly qualified. I liked my job with the American lawyers, often accompanying client's wives on shopping and sightseeing trips. I translated French correspondence, took French and English phone calls, and was fairly indispensable.

Ursula Andress, the original Bond girl in Dr. No, was one of the boss's clients and also his good friend. When she came swinging out of the elevator in a white silk blouse, with just a sliver of gossamer fabric between the world and those famous bouncing breasts, even I could see why men would happily give up just about anything to be in their proximity.

While focusing on my job, my life, my boyfriend, I tried not to think too much about what was going on at Chaban, nor how Father's romance was progressing. Maritee had left the job at our office and we rarely saw each other. It was all a bit confusing and I prayed Father would have the sense to continue visiting her in Paris, and not try to incorporate her in the kid's lives at Chaban.

On a hunch one day, I called Chaban. My sister Anne answered, sounding like Billy Goat Gruff.

"Hi" I said hopefully, "how are you?"

"Fine!" she grunted in a not very fine voice. My heart sank, we have always been able to read each other too well.

"Don't tell me Maritee is there," I whispered.

"Uh huh" my sister muttered in affirmative...

Oh my God, now what?! "Let me speak to Father" I said.

He came on the line, just bursting with enthusiasm and good will. "Hello darling, how are you, when are you coming to visit? Maritee is here and all the children **just love her**!"

There was nothing to say in the face of such blatant denial of the truth; Father had *invented* 'seeing what you want to see and nothing else'. He would ram this down the kid's throats and pretend everything was just perfect. He would not keep his lives separate for their sakes, he wanted everything and everyone he loved around him... and by God they all better pretend to like it.

A memorable trip spun out of this hurtful time. In his determination to knit this odd group together, father, now about forty five years young and custodian of *seven* children ranging in age from five to twenty, decided what we all needed to speed up the bonding process with his twenty two year old fiancée... Maritee now sporting a large, beautiful emerald and diamond ring… was a cruise in the Greek Islands.

Never one to go half way, he decreed that myself, Jenny, and our fifteen year old brother Peter could each bring a friend. He leased a beautiful 120ft sailboat, The Santa Maria, which met us at the dock in the Port of Piraeus.

Once onboard and sailing the seven seas, or the Greek ones at least, Jenny and her Raphael talked intense philosophy the entire time. No one could get a word in edgewise, they were in their own world. My very handsome Roland and I fought the entire trip… don't ask me about what, and Peter was in seventh heaven with a cute fourteen year old Belgian girl who had somehow talked her parents into letting her go sailing with us.

Roland and I fought so loudly up on the top deck once, screaming nonsense at each other just as we were coming into the serene port of Mykonos, that Jenny dropped her philosophy discussions long enough to run up behind Roland and hit him on the head with a hairbrush.

Stunned into silence, he and I were both were gifted with the irony of the scene…this perfect yacht gliding into this perfect port, spectators lining the quay to watch our magnificent entrance, probably thinking how lucky we were, and all we could think of was killing each other.

That evening at a restaurant Roland and I had another set-to. He got up from the table and huffed off into the night. Jacques, the lovely French professor who tutored the younger children and was a part of the family (who for some reason I have failed to mention until now), turned to me and said in French, *"Tu est vraiment mechante avec lui; va lui demander pardon!"* "You are so mean to him, go and tell him you are sorry."

"**You** go if you're so worried about him" I replied sharply.

So Jacques trotted off on his kind little legs to look for Roland. He found him walking along the beach in the dark towards the yacht. Catching up to him, he put an arm around his waist. His head barely reaching Roland's strong shoulders, Jacques murmured comforting things, probably telling him what a mean pig I was.

Roland didn't say much, Jacques told us later, just put his arm around Jacque's shoulder, squeezing him now and then and walking on quietly. It was only at the end of the beach, by the light of the dock that Jacques finally noticed he was arm in arm with a total stranger, a Greek stranger at that, more than happy to have the unexpected late night company.

Jacques took a page from my Gemini book and flew, getting back to the restaurant as we were leaving, just in time to convulse us with his story. Roland was asleep on the boat the whole time.

Although we fought in France, and we fought in Greece, and he even followed me back to California and fought with me there, Roland is still someone I call when I'm in Paris. He is always happy to see me, so many years later. Some things can not be explained.

Officially known as Thera, the Isle of Santorini is my favorite. We climbed up the one thousand steps to the top of this picturesque volcanic island (if there are less steps than that, it doesn't seem so when you are climbing them). We refused the little native donkeys that had been sent running down to give us a lift. They were so tiny it seemed heartless… so we climbed, step by hot dry step, to the top of the world.

Bright sunlight bounces off white walls everywhere you turn on these little streets. The church is magnificent in its simplicity… warm in its welcome. A tiny kitten abandoned by the curb is popped into Roland's pocket. So weak and shivering it is unlikely it will make it back down the thousand steps with us, let alone survive the perils of our yacht and its volatile inhabitants.

In a case like this I love being wrong. Once onboard the yacht, that dying little kitten turned into a roaring purring machine…a bit of food, a lot of love, and his entire little body started vibrating with the pitch of his happiness. You could hear him purring two cabins away. Fat, sassy and healthy at the end of the tumultuous Greek cruise, we were devastated to leave him behind, though glad to find him a home with kind cat lovers in Corfu.

At tiny Ios island my photographer's eye was entranced by the colorful fishing nets spread on the dock to dry. The daily ferry from Ios to a neighboring island was a phenomenon. A little flat-hulled vessel only big enough for ten people, it left the dock slowly, so slowly, with more than thirty passengers hanging on for dear life, the sea lapping perilously close to the top railing of the hull.

At every stop our yacht made, at every little village, there was a baker whose tiny shop smelled more fragrant than the last. *Psomi*. We couldn't get enough of that warm Greek bread, taking turns getting up at the first light of dawn to go off in search of it, tracking it down by its fragrance. 'Bread' and 'I love you' *s'agapo* were about the only Greek words I learned… *psomi* being hands down the most useful.

Then there was Delos. There is nothing on the little island of Delos except history; and two very worn, albeit large and magnificent stone lions facing the little harbor, guarding I know not what. According to legend, this tiny island with a land area of only 1.3 square miles, floated, until Zeus anchored it so Leto could give birth to the twins Apollo and Artemis.

The mythical twins were no longer in residence when we arrived. No one was. There may have been the odd goat, desperately seeking a blade of grass on that parched, barren piece of rock, but that was not enough to amuse our inquisitive and active group for three days, which is the amount of time we were stranded there.

The fierce September winds sprang up overnight, and the captain deemed it too dangerous to take the yacht out of the deserted little harbor until the winds dropped and he could slip out during a lull. At the end of three days, food supplies running low and tempers running high, the captain decided to make a run for it. He warned us the water would be rough and the going hard… which I for one did not like the sound of at all. Father of course was looking forward gleefully to the battle with nature.

Making the rounds of all the medicine chests and first aid kits onboard, I found a handful of Dramamine, anti-seasickness pills, and proceeded to take enough I thought, to let me sleep through the worst of the trip. There was no sensible Mother image on board, no one advised me against this, or if they did, I did not listen.

And so I slept, and slept, and slept…when I finally came around a day later, groggy, disoriented, thirsty and hungry, I headed to the upper deck. As I staggered against the teak walls of the corridor I realized the boat was blissfully still, we must be out of the storm. I wondered where everyone was, and why it was so quiet. Sticking my head out of the door to the main deck I saw a few family members watching me with strange, twisty looks on their faces, as if concealing some hidden mirth. My second glance took in the rocks behind them… *and those bloody lions!*

I had been asleep for twenty-four hours and the weather had been too rough to leave Delos.

That afternoon the weather broke. Wrapped in blankets and tarpaulins we dug ourselves into protected spots on deck, and headed off into the turbulent seas. The sleek vessel rode up the huge swells and slid down the troughs, extra large waves breaking over the bow with a crash. It *was* exhilarating I must say, much better than sleeping through it.

The trip ended in Corfu, where we grieved over giving up the little kitten, but had faith it would be happy with its new owners. Father somehow managed to get this hectic group back to France, where Maritee began her reign over Chaban. With a rather unsteady hand for the first few years.

My sister Jenny was hit with the worst of the shock of a new queen of the castle. From the age of fourteen she had supervised the running of the Chateau basically by herself, somehow managing to keep up her grades at school for the past two years while being substitute mother for all the younger kids… stressed to the point of having a nervous breakdown once at age sixteen, she burst into sobs in the middle of the courtyard, collapsing in hysterics.

As I mentioned, I had flown the coop. Jenny I am so very sorry, it was truly awful of me to leave all that to you, you were a rock to all of us. Please forgive me.

While Jenny was in charge, Father hadn't been able to sing her praises high enough. "Jenny did this and Jenny did that," and she deserved every morsel of that praise. Then without warning Jenny was out, and Maritee was in.

"Maritee did this today, Maritee did that today, isn't Maritee wonderful?"

Maritee smoked a small elegant wooden pipe with a long stem. Her favorite way of taunting the kids would be to lift her arse slightly off the chair saying to Father,

"I will be right back darling, I just need a little tobacco."

"Don't move darling, I'll get it," and Father would be off and running… Maritee barely containing her pleasure while the kids turned purple with frustrated anger.

I witnessed this myself on one of my lightning visits to Chaban. Father acting like a lovesick teenager, worshipping the ground she walked on. Maritee icily in control, ruthless, eyelashes fluttering in apparent devotion, taking over Father, taking over our home.

It made you want to puke, or contemplate murder. When she could not take it any more, Jenny went away quietly to Switzerland to visit Raphael and his family, where he proposed to her. Thank you Raphael for being there when Jenny needed you.

Jenny and Raphael had met soon after we moved to France. My mother was still in the picture when Father rented a ski chalet in Switzerland over the Christmas school vacation. Jenny broke her leg skiing, and she and mother stayed in the hospital while the leg healed, painfully swinging in the air with weights and trapezes for a month. The chalet owner, feeling badly about Jenny's accident, sent his two teenage sons to the hospital to cheer her up. There ensued some spirited rivalry between the boys, however Raphael remained steadfast, calling and corresponding months after Jenny's return to France, and won her heart.

Not sure she was ready to get married after the responsibilities and role of mother at Chaban, Jenny somehow ended up bicycling around India for six months to think things out. There she met a Catholic priest, and also met the Tibetan Lama father had spent time with. Between the two of them she was gently guided to a good decision. Jenny and Raphael married in the Catholic Church shortly after her return from India, and that has been perhaps the only enduring "happy marriage" I have had the privilege to witness.

Actually, I must correct myself. Despite the sparky currents shocking and upsetting others around their union, my father and his second wife eventually had what seemed like a happy, long and exciting life together.

They married in the South of France, traveling back to Chaban for a beautiful reception in the castle courtyard, followed by a Benson style picnic. Carriages loaded with breads and hams, quilts and cushions, wine and fruits, pastries and cakes, all convening at the chosen spot by a stream, under a shady oak tree, down in my favorite beautiful valley. The ladies wore Renaissance dresses with flowers in their hair, the men were in ruffled shirts, and someone played an instrument under a nearby tree. Father missed his calling, he would have made a great choreographer.

Maritee soon had the first of her three lovely daughters, and began to feel more at ease at Chaban. She never did appreciate the great stones and forests as we did however, and often longed for 'a smaller place she could call her own', perhaps something that was not so imbibed with her husband's previous life.

Father and Maritee went to India together a year or two after their wedding, and returned with a small group of Tibetan lamas and monks eager to accept their hospitality and refuge on our land in the Dordogne. Translators and followers soon arrived in large numbers, and for a few months the whole entourage lived in the Castle.

Their comings and goings were unsettling for the younger children, for it was not unusual to turn a corner inside the castle, deep in thought, on an important errand - or even an unimportant errand, and run smack into a smiling lama in a saffron robe, lost in the cavernous rooms of the castle.

Until the day the Tibetans decided to take up father's offer to make France their permanent home. Suddenly the castle emptied and the saffron robes took up residence a mile down the road in the stone farmhouse father turned over to them. People from far and near began arriving to be in the presence of these enlightened Teachers. They stayed to help renovate the farm buildings, to shop and cook for the lamas. Several of the younger men and women built A-frame meditation huts for themselves nearby; often leaving friends and family stunned by their choice to live such a contemplative life near the lamas and far from home.

We will come back to the adventures of Tibetan lamas and monks in the French countryside, but first we must go to the Bahamas for the conception of my daughter.

GREEK GODS AND TIBETAN PRAYER FLAGS

I met Genevieve's Dad at the Poolside Restaurant of the secluded Lyford Cay Club, tucked away on the western tip of New Providence Island, only a few miles, but a million light years away from the chaos of downtown Nassau. Introductions were made and I found myself looking up into the slate green eyes of a Greek god. Tall, lean, tan and muscular. A warm handshake and a flash of something electric in those eyes.

Over lunch it was inevitable I fall in love, or in lust at any rate. He was gorgeous, well mannered, well spoken, articulate, in charge… and fascinated by me. He would have been devilishly difficult to resist under any circumstances, and right now, on a two week leave of absence from a stagnant live-in relationship in Paris, my middle name was 'vulnerable'. This exotic place, this compelling man's instant powerful feelings for me, this was life! I was ready for the fairy tale… the Knight on a White Horse.

Paris had been gray and rainy for months. The beautiful stone buildings were totally devoid of their usual light and luster, the Parisians were depressed and grumpy, and even the tight little espresso coffees served in cafés everywhere at all hours seemed to have lost their kick.

The transition time of a nine-hour flight found me scurrying for sunglasses in a startlingly different landscape. Here the air was bright and sweet, humming with unseen insects and poignantly colored butterflies, the lush foliage and explosions of tropical flowers even more beautiful than the splashy TV ads promised.

The heat in the air and in those green eyes enveloped me, seduced me, made me forget the cold days and bleak gray stones of Paris as if they never existed. Where the French relationship had been comfortable but not particularly passionate, this new love was full of romance and desire, full of promises of Forever … and angelic children.

In the throes of this magic encounter straight out of a romance novel, it did not strike warning chords with me that my green-eyed hunk… a dead ringer for Tom Selleck at age thirty, had only four months previously left his second wife and a good job in New York, and would not speak of her; that his father had died of a heart attack just ten days before we met; that his mother was a heavy drinker at the time and expected him to continue living with her in the comfortable house in Lyford Cay. A shrink would have had a field day with that information…I blindly ignored it.

Ensconced in my beautiful cottage on Cable Beach, reveling as I was in the tropical gardens, in the swimming pool on the terrace just a few feet across the sand from the turquoise Bahamian waters … seeing clearly was the last thing on my mind. *Au contraire*, with this romantic, very romantic interest so abruptly in my life, I thought perhaps I had fainted and woken up in my very own niche in Paradise.

The main house was aptly named *La Playa*, The Beach. A stunning tribute to colonial architecture, it was a white, wedding cake house, nestled right on the pristine sand. Two stories of immense rooms, bedrooms with balconies overlooking the sea, libraries, music rooms, sweeping staircases… not exactly your average beach house. Friends living in London had snapped it up for a song when the American Embassy put it up for sale, complete with sterling silverware and exquisite china for intimate little dinner parties of thirty or so, the magnificent dining room table and carved armchairs designed to accommodate just that number.

When asked how it came about that my life took a turn from Paris to the Bahamas, I remember the standing invitation from Christian and Felicity to visit them in the Bahamas; and the day I grasped it like a lifeline, unable to get through one more dreary, gray day in Europe… the year the rain drizzled for six months in Paris, from December to July.

* * * * *

Preferring the relative cool of a London summer to the heat of Nassau, Christian and Felicity had no plans to visit until October, and told me to enjoy myself in their house, adding as an afterthought, "You might find it a bit hot." Foolishly, I presumed they were referring to the climate.

Their driver and butler, a lovely oldstyle Bahamian gentleman, met me at Nassau airport. We drove along the coast to the wedding cake house. I fell in love with it immediately, and the gardens, and the sea, and the Greek god soon thereafter.

Despite warnings all my life about the inherent dangers of sunbathing, the first few days were spent soaking up the sun. Years ago I made the choice to live a short tan life rather than a long pallid one. God so far has been kind to me.

Suddenly having a change of heart, my friends said they would fly in from London a few days later, and throw a big party over the weekend to introduce me to the *Who's Who* of Nassau. By then I had banished my Paris pallor and acquired a golden glow. Thus I met the Baroness, who introduced me to her tennis partner over lunch at Lyford Cay Club the next day…the Marlboro Man in yachting attire who was to become Genevieve's dad.

We spent an idyllic few weeks together, swimming, boating, talking, 'courting'. I called Paris and said something to the effect that, "I won't be back until September, and then only to collect my belongings, I'll be getting married and moving to the Bahamas."

"Well!" Paris said, "Blow me down with a feather!" An outlandish expression, rendered even more so coming from a solidly built American lawyer.

Gen's future dad and I spent hours exploring far away deserted beaches, collecting shells from secret coves, feeding wild iguanas; three foot long prehistoric lizards, their snapping teethblades a hazard to friendly fingers offering food in return for a photo. No signs posted, "Be wary of fingermunchers." No flapping paper debris, no footprints in the sand but ours. No sign of life at all other than the dinosaurs… sole residents of this little cay forgotten by time.

Back in the people world, lunch at the hamburger stand on the dunes of the Club's spectacular beach was a casual affair, with the 26ft Sea Ray anchored in the gentle surf of the bay just a few steps away. If something fancier was desired in the culinary department, clothes were thrown over bathing suits and we dined at the Poolside Restaurant, forever the romantic place Where We First Met.

On day Ten of this idyllic life, my knight did not drop me off on the beach in front of La Playa as had been his custom, pulling the boat into five inches of water for my convenience, jumping overboard and gracefully lifting me over the bow and onto the beach with a hug and a kiss. Waving goodbye, with tanned muscles bulging he would push the boat back into deeper water, spring lithely onto the dive platform, climb into the boat, take the controls, and be off with a mighty roar of engines. My hero.

No, on this day we glided quietly past the yachts lined up in the Lyford Cay Marina, and into one of the myriad wide canals that pass in front of houses of the rich and famous. We had cruised through here several times before, and I did not think much of it, lounging back in the copilot's comfy chair, feet up on the control panel, chatting about this and that. My hair was bedraggled from a day's swimming, my bikinied body half naked and lightly dusted in fine pink sand from playing in the surf at the edge of a remote beach. Had I any choice in the matter of an appropriate moment to meet Mother, this would not have made the list.

Meet her I did. The boat pulled up at the dock right in front of her house, the sudden realization of what was happening dawning on me only when a diminutive redheaded woman sailed out from the house in full regalia… long flowing Pucci gown, every hair in place, discreet but impressive jewelry, perfect makeup. Across the lawn and out onto the dock she sailed, where my beloved said without further ado, "Hello Mother, this is Bernadette."

Too shocked to kill him on the spot, I did my best to look dignified, shook the outstretched hand, and dived for a towel to cover the offending body that had so obviously been off cavorting with her son… leaving her miserably home alone.

After a quick shower, I changed into shorts and a T-shirt, items that could just as easily have been put on before the unexpected First Encounter. Now it was too little, too late. Mother was greatly annoyed, that was obvious. So uptight her lips could barely pry themselves apart to speak. Although a master at bluffing my way with confidence and European *savoir faire* through most situations, this one left me breathless. I had been led into ambush by the man who was supposed to protect me.

Clothed now, less naked but not much more comfortable, I had to endure Mother sniffing down her nose at me, doing her best to be polite, wanting to strangle her son. One of the rare thoughts we both agreed on.

It was a bad beginning to a prickly relationship. Meeting on even turf, both of us elegantly dressed and composed would have provided some sport for both of us; this was shooting ducks in a gallery.

* * * * *

So lost was I in my fairytale romance, love seemed to conquer all. Despite this 'first encounter with Mother' hiccup, my knight and I, his armor now slightly tarnished, embarked on a trip to France to meet my family. Arriving in Paris, my love allotted me just two hours to pack up two years of belongings from the beautiful apartment in the Champs de Mars overlooking the Eiffel Tower, the apartment I had so recently shared with the Paris boyfriend.

My hero paced beside the car three stories below, thus assuring that no meeting with the 'ex' would take place. As I hurriedly threw treasured bits and pieces into suitcases, making irrevocable choices in the bat of an eye, I noted bemusedly to myself that this worked out to be one hour of packing for each year of living here..

Thinking it "cute" that my new love was jealous and didn't want me to have anything to do with the past boyfriend, I let him have his way. Later I would see the folly of such a questionable beginning to our life together.

My navy blue Lancia with its beautiful creamy leather seats was waiting for us near the apartment in an underground garage, where I had left it before my precipitous flight to the Bahamas.

I loved the aroma of leather wafting around me, perhaps because it evokes memories of my early beginnings in Father's bomber jacket, or the hours spent in the western saddles of my childhood. I loved even more hearing the car start on the first try, eager as I was to be out of Paris and onto the curving country roads that offered more of a challenge to the car's superlative handling.

The drive from Paris to Chaban can take anywhere from six to eight hours, depending on the time of departure, 5a.m. being the best, 8a.m. the worst. At play is also whether one is enjoying the scenery, or just 'getting there' which involves speeds of 100 mph whenever roads permit.

Once out of the perimeters of Paris, it is a very beautiful drive. I particularly love the area of Sologne, where pheasants, deer and even the odd wild boar are likely to dash across the road in front of you, inexplicably desperate not to miss something on the other side.

And the great fields of sunflowers. Oh how I loved those sunflowers, and how my little daughter would love them one day, although I could not foresee this as we sped by fields and fields of them. Flowers tall as a pretty woman, masses of them stretching as far as the eye can see.

They are called *Tournesol* in France, and throughout the day will turn their lovely yellow faces to follow the sun; thus a photo of a field taken in the morning light, and another taken in the afternoon, will show the flowers facing a completely different direction.

This time the stunningly beautiful drive from Paris to Chaban was marred by the unpleasant memory of an overnight stop in a small, quaint hotel along the bank of a small river. A beautiful, romantic spot, where the possibility of soaking together in a huge bathtub should have been ecstasy, particularly given how rare it is to find a large tub in a French country hotel. Yet there I soaked alone, puzzled and angry. My love's sinewy length stretched out on the bed on top of the pretty quilted eiderdown, his handsome face gazing at the ceiling in a sulk. He refused to join me in the tub, he refused to talk to me. He was lost in his sulk.

Happy memories should have been in the making, yet there he lay, preferring to mull over some slight I must have incurred, some infraction he didn't want to expound on.

The details of the sulk escape me, if indeed I was ever made privy to them, but the memory of the frustration lingers. He cheered up at some point however, again for reasons unknown to me, and upon arriving at the Castle we had a wonderful, warm visit with my father. The men hugged, and both shed tears.

My mother is not in the picture at this time, having gone off to London for the infamous weekend with the boyfriend. The weekend that precipitated a drama far worse than any of us could possibly have imagined.

My love and I went to visit the Tibetan lamas in residence on the estate. They were still living in the original stone farmhouse father had given them, only now it was transformed into a thriving Tibetan Center, complete with a spacious reception area offering books, videos, class schedules, and flyers detailing an impending visit to the Center by the Dalai Lama. A meeting between the Marlboro Man and several of the lamas was not met with the ridicule I might have expected from this man I knew so little about. In fact he seemed to find the brief encounter fascinating.

We returned to Nassau bolstered with father's blessing. We didn't get around to choosing a wedding date right away however, and probably would have dawdled on without a plan for ages. The thought of organizing a wedding with both families present, deciding who of my huge and scattered family to invite, the travel distances and expenses, the accommodations etc; I could go on ad nauseum, as anyone knows who has gone through one or several marriages. This was one area neither of us really wanted to tackle.

Christian and Felicity flew in from London unexpectedly and invited us to lunch. Somewhere between the salmon and the orange soufflé, Christian said out of the blue, "If you get married this Saturday, we will take care of the wedding, the flowers, the catering, everything… we'll have it here in the garden, then you'll fly with us in the jet to our ranch in Texas for your honeymoon!"

Well that was an offer we could not refuse. We were married on a warm breezy day in January, in the gardens of La Playa, seven months from the day we met, in such a rush there was no time to invite my family, which I later regretted. Friends were in abundance, my love's Mother floated and greeted, managing to look lovely while barely suppressing thoughts of murder. (Her son's? Mine? Both of us?).

The wedding was quite simply divine. I swept down the graceful curving staircase to meet the Baron, husband of the lovely lady who introduced me to my Knight. On his arm I made my entrance through a flowering yellow and white archway to the Garden, where our friends were gathered in soft rays of January sunlight, their faces a smiling blur to me as I looked for the one face that mattered.

We met. The transfer from the Baron's arm to the groom was a subtle shift that would forever change my life, for better and for worse. The elegant Minister said the words we had given him, had prepared together, words from John Denver's song *Perhaps Love* which brought tears to our eyes at the time; words I can not now recall.

We signed the registry, mingled with friends, had a perfect lunch, cut a perfect cake, the first one like it ever seen in the Bahamas. It was copied from my memories of a French wedding cake, a two foot tower of cascading honey colored creampuffs, held together with clear caramel and scattered with tiny rosebuds tucked in here and there, peeking out, as only cheeky tiny rosebuds can do. A traditional slice in the top tier of the pyramid, then mounds of creamy centered caramel profiterolles piled on every plate.

Wedding photos show such love in our eyes, misty tears, perfect harmony. Where does that love and emotion go when it goes? Does another happy wedding party grab it? Does it hover above us waiting for the right circumstances to reappear? Or does it mutate, turning into something ugly and painful… I would like to know.

And Yes, we took their private jet to Texas, and Yes, they came and stayed at the ranch with us… and Yes, this was where I first noticed my beloved could spend hours sulking and not talking to me, but could perch happily on a kitchen counter and chat most amicably with my friends.

From day one of our honeymoon, the Marlboro Man and I found getting along together on a daily basis so different from our idyllic courtship.

I am a Gemini, he is a Scorpio, so perhaps we should have read up on each other's personalities. I did not like nor understand his long glum days; he could not stand my cheerful chatting and insatiable curiosity. We muddled through our honeymoon, came home to live with his mother in Lyford Cay and began to deal with real, or unreal, life.

It became evident in the first five minutes of our return to Nassau after the Texas honeymoon, and I use the term loosely, that we had to find a place of our own. His mother had not wanted her darling to be married again, had expected him to replace the husband she had just lost, and did not understand why he had let her down like this.

Impatient to start our life together, just the two of us, I was not particularly interested in her desperate need to be part of our lives, and was certainly not always patient or kind. There are some things in life we wish we had done differently.

Quite soon we moved out of her house in Lyford Cay and into a townhouse in Cable Beach, not far from where we were married. The townhouse complex was also owned by my love's mother. She had properties all over the place, and had worked hard to acquire them. For twenty years she owned and managed an elegant woman's clothing boutique, specializing in Emilio Pucci designs and accessories at a time when the great designer was alive. She knew him personally from numerous visits to his atelier in Italy.

About the time she and I met so infortuitously, the bloom had begun to fade on the demand for the colorful designs that had delighted the Lyford Cay crowd for many years. Traveling to Europe in search of new designs without her husband did not appeal to her and interest in the business began to wane.

My new husband, (or her son, which was he? It didn't occur to either of us that he could perhaps be both) went to work with the bank Christian had started in Nassau. I jumped into redecorating the townhouse we lived in, with Mother's approval. As soon as it was finished I moved on to the five adjoining apartments. Most of the tenants were thrilled with the results and had no objection to the increased rents, and the few who moved out were replaced immediately at the new rate. Thus Mother's rental income from the townhouses was doubled within a few months of my becoming her unwanted daughter-in-law.

We were on our own for two months in the townhouse. In short order she leased her Lyford Cay house out to friends and moved into the townhouse next door to us.

My husband and I did manage to have some great and wonderful moments in the beginning, and I will still tell anyone who asks that the first ten days after I met my knight were the best ten days of my life.

I began helping out in Mother's boutique. The clothes were beautiful quality and it was a pleasure finding the perfect way to showcase the European designs for her clients. A phone call out of the blue announced that my sister Wendy was coming to visit me from Hong Kong. She was working there with a then unheard of designer, Diane Freis. The samples Wendy brought with her to Nassau were striking in design, and the fabrics were to die for. Organizing a Hong Kong to Bahamas shipping system, we soon filled the shop with dozens of Diane Freis Originals, each one a unique design, a different fabric, an unusual cut, and one more beautiful than the next.

When the ladies of Lyford Cay discovered that the fabrics flowed and felt like silk, that they could be folded to wisps of nothing for traveling, and could be machine washed with no ill effects, the stampede was on.

The designs danced out the door for the next five years until I was fired, out of the shop, and out of my marriage… although I believe it was in the reverse order.

* * * * *

Upon setting eyes on me that first blissful lunch at Lyford Cay Club, my knight had confidently foreseen children appearing within nine months and one minute of our marriage. No little ones had showed signs of materializing by the end of the first year, when we combined a business trip to Europe, clients for him, fashion designs for me. A stopover in the Dordogne was on the agenda, we would stay at the castle to visit my family, now his family too.

We rested briefly after the train ride from Paris to the country, my husband was then adamant about strolling down the lane to see the lamas again. It seems that on our first visit to France he had taken to heart the few minutes spent with them. Impressed with stories he heard regarding their wisdom and powers of healing, he now wanted their opinion on the best way to kick start our family.

My sister Heather lived nearby, and was asked by Lama Gendun to translate for us. One of three siblings who spent years studying the Tibetan language and spiritual teachings, she often traveled with the Lamas to Paris, translating Tibetan to either French or English at official functions, and a few years later would co-author a book with the Dalai Lama. Her fluency in the Tibetan language was a rare accomplishment, and her interpretations would be faultless, yet this was the one sister with whom I did not get on particularly well. It made me uncomfortable knowing she would be privy to questions of such a personal nature.

Lama Gendun soon put us all at ease however, and when my husband asked him,

"How many children will we have?" He roared with laughter and said,

"What do you think I am, a fortune teller!?"

He showed us the lovely rose colored prayer beads he held in his hands and said, "I have never been to the Bahamas, yet I can *feel your lives* in these beads, they are made from the coral of your country."

This smiling wise man had spent three decades of his sixty years in isolated meditations in the mountains of his homeland Tibet, before being ripped from his country by the Chinese. Escaping with his quiet, fragile life, tossed unceremoniously on the good will of peoples of strange and varied countries, he finally found a home in France that, while unable to replace his own, met at least in terms of peacefulness and beauty, some of his old comforts…For this my father is to be remembered.

On this tranquil mountaintop, in this sweet part of France or "La Douce France" as the Dordogne is sometimes called, he was happy to share his wisdom with us in the good humored, tranquil and warm way that is a Tibetan wiseman's trademark.

It did not surprise me at all to find a Tibetan Lama sitting in a French farmhouse using prayer beads made from Bahamian coral.

Lama Gendun gave my husband a mysterious fertility mantra to hum about a billion times a day, and blessed a beautiful prayer flag before giving it to us to fly in front of our house in the Bahamas.

Tibetan prayer flags are pieces of art. Long strips of gauzy, light fabric are dyed in a variety of colors (usually yellow, blue, white, or sienna red) then cut to about ten inches in width, by six to ten feet long. Prayers are then printed the length of the fabric in black ink, using ancient wooden printing blocks. When these flags are hung from tall posts, fastened top and bottom like a sail, the prayers are carried away on the winds, to places where prayers are heard.

Often several tall poles with different colored flags festoon one garden or property. At the Tibetan Center, flags line both sides of the long walkway, enveloping in peace and prayer everyone who enters.

Back in Nassau, the combination of our deep red prayer flag flying over the turquoise Bahamian seas, and the devout repetition of the mantras by my husband created powerful results. Scoff if you will, we saw Lama Gendun in early April... Genevieve was born January 20 of the following year, ten months after our visit to Lama Gendun.

THE WATUSI

You never saw such a beautiful baby. Smiling, happy, the apple of her father's eye. So tiny he could cradle her with one big hand, carrying her about the house everywhere he went. Home from work early just for the pleasure of gazing at her while she slept, Daddy had her in the tranquil turquoise Bahamas water with him before she was six months old. When she was barely one he was tossing her in the air above his head shouting, "I love you!" and his grin and her peal of laughter would warm my heart.

Those moments held me together, and tore me apart.

In the months before Gen was born, nightmares of being alone in an empty desert had terrified me. Running everywhere in the thick, hot sand, frantically searching for something or someone. Running in a silent vacuum... running, running, always alone... searching for what? Waking with heart pounding to find I was not alone, but had a husband sleeping next to me... then the numbing realization that this brought me no comfort, did not make me feel one bit less alone.

I couldn't bring myself to discuss this dread with him. How do you say such a thing to a person and expect them to be comforting? I did not know that in a good marriage you should be able to do just that. Didn't know that my inability to speak was in itself a barometer of how our marriage was not all it should be.

I am told, having never experienced it for myself, that in a solid relationship such fears can be thrown into the open for discussion, evaluation and ideally resolution, without horrible arguments and more pain resulting on both sides. I did not know that the magic of a good marriage can be hidden in the warmth that comes from giving comfort when things are difficult; that the magic can explode into the heart-thumping joy of shared happiness when things are great. To my great regret, I know not of what I speak.

My sister Jenny living in Switzerland would have been an immense help had I but thought to turn in that direction. We were not as close as we are now, or I would have seen the obvious; she managed to guide her marriage through the ups and downs of bringing five children into the world, while integrating her husband's transition from busy medical student to much sought after doctor.

So busy was Raphael at one point in their lives, he could not find time to enjoy life with his family on weekends. Exhausted and plagued with headaches from researching cures and giving hope all day, every day, to people other doctors deemed terminal, for this was the field in which he found his calling, there was nothing left for himself or his family.

A handsome, lovely, enlightened couple, they gradually rearranged their lives to make time to take vacations together in the Swiss mountains, or a few days in the gabled stone house left to her in France by Father. My wise and patient sibling was able to lead her husband to see the wisdom of molding his strenuous schedule into a less stressful one, to take on a shorter list of patients, to allow a bit more time for each one and still have time for himself and their family.

Now they have a life. They laugh, walk, talk, picnic, swim, and bike together, often with their numerous children and sometimes just quiet moments to themselves. Raphael is a cycling fanatic. Now he has time for his passion; racing up and down those twisting Swiss mountain roads on weekends; zipping along the country roads of France during his well deserved holidays. He is a younger, stronger, more vital man than a few years ago, and visibly happier with his more manageable schedule and serene home life. Gentle guidelines held them together through the proverbial thick and thin.

Not thinking to seek help in that direction, I was alone in Paradise, now a deserted wasteland void of any source of sensible advice or uplifting ideas.

Nassau is a small town, nothing is sacred, nothing could be said that the whole town wouldn't hear. There was not one safe person to speak to, no attempt could be made to release this torment inside… no one to ask, "Why am I so afraid?"

Left with only myself to talk to, repeating the same questions yet hearing no answers, the months before my baby was born were passed in conflicting tides of great happiness, and terrifying uncertainties.

In the last month or so, my svelte body bulked up to someone I did not recognize; someone who had to waddle from point A to point B, someone who, perhaps in an oversensitive and paranoid state, saw her husband casting longing looks at the attractive redhead working at his mother's Boutique. Someone who thought she saw him putting his hands on that voluptuous body as he passed by a little closer than necessary, someone who kept hearing rumors that he also had a fancy for the tall brunette working in his office across the street. Rumors? Imaginings? The truth? Only he and they will ever know for sure.

Having no one close at hand to talk to during the pregnancy was really not good. The doctor recommended to us as the best on the

Island was a very large, intimidating Nigerian man with a flashy gold Rolex on his wrist that no gloves or gown were meant to hide.

This doctor was not a person I felt comfortable submitting my questions to. You were lucky if the nurse called you into his office within two hours of your appointment, and luckier still to be given five minutes of his time. I went to see him as rarely as possible.

And I was terrified. Hadn't I decided I didn't want to have children? Hadn't my brothers and sisters been through so much after our parents split… no more laughter, only confusion and pain for years… that I thought it better not to have kids at all?

On top of being overly concerned that the baby inside me might not be well, might not have the required number of fingers and toes, might not come out right at all… it now seemed that every well intentioned Bahamian woman had some bit of local folklore to impart to me. No matter how unlikely their tale, *once in my head how to get the images out?*

Thus in my fourth month when I was told, *"Never put your hands up over your head or the baby's umbilical cord will get wrapped around its neck"*… that was the last time I put my hands past my shoulders for five months. Couldn't reach up into a cupboard, didn't dare put my arms around my husband's neck, could barely brush my hair or get into a sweater. Knowing it was ridiculous didn't help one bit.

Yes, I had my beautiful baby in Nassau, in a very up to date private hospital that turned out to be excellent. The doctor however, did not deserve his exalted reputation, and was in fact responsible for my decision in the days following the 'happy event' not to ever go through the experience again… thank you very much!

I won't bore you with the gory details, suffice to say that after my husband spent six hours fanning me with a file folder so I could breath, I told him him in no uncertain terms, "I don't want to do this anymore, stop everything!" He just fanned harder. The doctor dashed in for a quick peek in the seventh hour. He looked at his watch (the famous Rolex) and said,

"I have a cesarean to do down the hall in fifteen minutes so PUSH."

When this did not immediately have the desired effect, he picked up a scalpel and performed an episiotomy without any mention of his intentions, tossed the baby to a nearby nurse, then proceeded to sew me up with no anesthetic at the precise moment I should have been basking in the thrill of my baby's new life, reveling in the joy and peace of holding my 'precious bundle' for the first time.

My husband had to hold me down, and almost fainted from the screaming. Sorry, a couple of gory details seem to have snuck in there despite my promises.

During the months after our beautiful baby was born, the nightmares turned into frightening 'daymares' of suicide.

Why couldn't I speak out about these black, black thoughts? Why couldn't I trust my husband with this burden that was weighing down my life, sucking the joy out of it? Why was it so much easier to lash out at small annoyances than face these fears with him, why did we seem to be bringing out the worst in each other instead of the best?

So many questions and so few answers.

With no method, plan, or wisdom to guide me during either our marriage or the breakup, I was flying by the seat of my pants within a narrow viewpoint devoid of any spirituality. Emotions were flapping in the wind, common sense was left in another lifetime. Is it any wonder that it is my lot to be left with the gnawing guilt of handling badly this very crucial point in my life.

Not being a fan of 'cheer me up' drugs, and no discreet friends in sight to help me get a grip, with my family far away in Europe busy with their own lives, and my husband oblivious to my inner torment… there was nowhere to turn. Certainly no good advice forthcoming from his mother, who still let me know at every opportunity that her son had promised he wouldn't marry again after leaving his 'beautiful and talented' second wife in New York… that he, "came back to Nassau to live with her, his mother."

She reminded me her husband had died just ten days before I met her son, "and it was unfortunate, terrible timing, that I had come to the Bahamas just when she needed him so much." Certainly no help coming from that quarter… and with God forgotten in my anguish, our marriage was doomed.

* * * * *

When Genevieve was seven months old we accompanied her Dad to London on a business trip. I did seek help then, making an appointment with a well known Harley Street specialist recommended by a London friend.

I told this doctor in his splendid office that I had a wonderful, handsome husband, (he looked like a young Tom Selleck at the time) who loved me very much, a beautiful baby, and a life in a sunny Island that most people only dream of.

"So why?" I asked him, "Do I spend three hours of every day playing out different scenarios on how to kill myself without my family thinking it was anything but an accident?"

"If I put cans of gasoline in the back of the green car left us by my husband's father, and rammed it into a tree, would that work? Would the car and I be devoured enough by the flames so the gas cans would not leave a clue? What is the matter with me?"

This paltry excuse for a doctor, Ferguson was his name, looked at me and said, "My dear, you are far too attractive to be thinking of killing yourself; here, take these pills twice a day for a year."

I was thirty six years old, coping with the confinement of a first marriage and a seven month old baby… after years of flitting around the globe free as a lark. Yet this Incompetent never mentioned the words Postpartum Depression. I had never heard those words myself, or it had never clicked as something that would apply to me. He never said, "Yes, there is something wrong with you, your hormones are like Whirling Dervishes and need to be put into balance."

Just a vial of anti-depressants. No grain of comfort or hope, not even the most basic "Don't worry, this is quite common after having a baby, just a bad patch to get through together with your husband, I'll tell him how he can help."

Simple words that would have put our lives back in perspective. A missed chance to save a marriage; to give a child the gift of growing up with two parents, feeling secure and loved, instead of years of rejection and a sense of loss that took years to overcome..

The anti-depressants put me into a quasi coma. A nightmare of pulling myself out of sucking sands and oozing mud. I preferred my own nightmares, and threw out the pills. Things did not get any better, they went from bad to worse. Two years later we separated, Gen was not yet three.

* * * * *

Genevieve has not come home. Night has definitely fallen, it is pitch black outside, and the brilliant moon of Hopetown is hidden behind dark clouds.

We have very few rules in this house of mother and daughter, 'Be polite, help out when you can, leave a return time on our message pad when you go out, or check in by five p.m. to advise of plans for the evening'.

Tonight there are no plans, there is only darkness, and I am assailed anew with guilt. Bowled over by what this only child of mine has had to endure at the hands of the textbook wicked stepmother, and an absent, "I'm very busy now with my new family" father since the age of three.

In an obviously misguided attempt to discover why our five-year marriage wasn't working, I asked my husband to move out for a few weeks, thinking it was not good for Genevieve to see us arguing, that with a bit of distance between us he and I could find a way to resolve our grievances.

Within a month of being out on his own, lonely for family life but not wanting to face our problems squarely, or at all, Gen's Daddy allowed himself to be engulfed by a very tall, attractive Bahamian woman whom I called, among other things, The Watusi. She should be pleased… to my knowledge the Watusi are a very tall, elegant and noble tribe, renowned for their great warriors.

I've gotten ahead of myself, bear with me.

Several months before moving out, Gen's Dad had started jogging to lose the few pounds he had packed on over the last couple of years of married life. We both liked to cook. He would dash out immediately after work every evening, just when Gen wanted to spend time with him, then return so sweaty and exhausted he could barely talk, let alone play games with her.

She watched these comings and goings stoically enough for several weeks, then began hearing her Dad say how pleased he was with the weight he was losing. As he leaned over the couch to give her a kiss goodbye on his way out one evening, she said quite articulately for a two year old, "Daddy why do you have to go jogging now that you have lost weight?" A simple question really, one that meant, "Why can't you stay and play with me?"

Her Dad looked stunned, and when it was obvious he could think of nothing to say, I began to explain, "Punkin, once you start exercising, it feels good and you want to continue doing it." Suddenly he came alive, jumping all over me in his loud bullying voice, "Kids only need yes or no answers, what are you going on with all this philosophical rubbish for!" It was my turn to be stunned.

Soon thereafter a 'pre-owned' gold BMW arrived from the States. No, it was not a lovely surprise for me, he made it quite clear he did not want me driving it. In September Gen and I went to Europe by ourselves to see my family, while Dad stayed in Nassau. As the transatlantic telephone calls had been less than satisfying while Gen and I were away, I asked him to move out of the house for a couple of months, thinking if we weren't living in the same house we would be able to get a better perspective and be able to sort out the problems in our marriage. In all fairness, before packing he did say if he left he would not be back. I just needed him out so I could think, and didn't 'hear' him.

He moved out, going to live with a neighbor… until the Watusi showed up at his office a few weeks later on the recommendation of a friend, to advise him on new drapes… I have always thought she must have given good drape.

With two children under five by previous relationships and barely making ends meet with a job at a travel company, the Watusi moved him into her apartment and her life as quick as a flash, then proceeded to get pregnant two months later… just two months shy of our daughter's third birthday.

This crafty woman was not about to let her handsome catch nor his trendy gold BMW escape from her clutches…she drove that car up and down Nassau ten times a day, waving and shouting to all her friends, happy as a pig in a poke. A woman who not only knew what she wanted, but how to get it.

She now had a man to take care of her children and provide them all with a better life. She knew that he wanted more children, and becoming pregnant so quickly was not a risk to her; she did so in the certainty that he would not leave her with a child on the way.

She immediately established he was not to go near me, our house, or Genevieve, terrified he might spend time with his daughter and come to his senses. She was as good as a bloodhound, invariably tracking him down by phone within ten minutes of any impromptu visit to Gen… with an apparently irresistible reason why he had to go home to her right away.

She hit the nail on the head in a whiny note to him I saw on his desk (it is a woman's gift to be adept at reading upside down). "Honey you are the best thing that ever happened to me, please don't leave me."

Compared to a wife who blamed him for our mutual unhappiness, not knowing or caring enough to seek professional family counseling, or at the very least a competent medical evaluation for me, thrashing around blindly for two and a half years after our daughter's birth in the throes of an undiagnosed "post baby" depression, this new woman's grateful attitude must have seemed heavensent to him.

Genevieve's Dad now in another woman's home. No time to work out anything, no time for Genevieve to see her Father more than fleetingly, and then furtively, against the pregnant girlfriend's orders.

When asking my husband to leave for a few weeks, it never crossed my mind that Genevieve would cry every night for one solid hour, for one solid year, asking, "Why isn't my Daddy coming home?" I swear it did not ever come up and slap me in the face until it was too late.

I thought she would be fine alone with me until he and I could work out our differences. It was in the back of my mind that we would find our love again, that he would move back in with us, life would be fun again, without the inexplicable tensions and the useless, spiteful arguments. This was not to be.

No matter what our differences, no matter what effort it took, had I really understood the turmoil and grief that lay ahead for my daughter, and thereby for me, I would have found a way to resolve those differences come hell or high water.

I had heard so often, even had firsthand proof with my own little brothers during my parent's traumatic split, that it was always the children who suffer most in the midst of parental disharmony.

Yet blindly, stubbornly, selfishly, I forged ahead, crucifying our beautiful daughter because we adults weren't 'happy enough'. In fairness to myself, I did make attempts to regroup. After several distressing weeks of seeing how very much Gen missed her Dad, after realizing there was a possibility he had no plans to work things out, I have a painful recollection of actually begging him to stay with us until Gen was five, reasoning that if we could stay together as a family for just two more years, she would have time for at least a glimpse of two-parent family life. Perhaps time to amass enough memories to store and sustain her through the tough times to come. Perhaps even time for us to get the magic back.

He replied coldly, "It's better to split now while she is little."

Hindsight is a great teacher but a source of vast sadness and regret. Surely I could have cleared my mind throughout those first weeks of separation enough to focus on the only important fact; Genevieve deserved and needed her two parents.

When a parent dies, and the other is left to soldier on alone, that is a different tragedy for both child and spouse, a different sense of loss. But a father who is down the road with another family…that leaves a sense of abandonment and betrayal that has to be overcome every day in a million small ways.

Surely I could have summoned the strength and the appropriate measure of conciliation and dignity needed to get through to her Dad. Surely I could have found *someone* to talk with us, to mediate, to bring us back to the positive things in our lives.

Why had I presumed we would have time to work things out? Why didn't it occur to me he might meet someone else right away? I honestly thought we would both use the time apart to get a grip on the real issues, would spend the time learning to be civil, perhaps even kind to one another again. Where did my thinking go so wrong?

When imparting the dreaded message years ago to my little brothers that our Mum was not coming back, little more than a child myself, I thought then that I knew all about pain. I could not know how much worse the pain is when you are a parent, and you are watching your own child suffer.

Little Gen waiting for the telephone to ring, then seeing her face crumple when it wasn't her Dad, when it wasn't the invitation or a promise to visit she needed so badly… feeling the black hole in my heart and stomach at the realization there is nothing, nothing to be done in that moment to melt the blow. The stomach sinks, I don't know where it goes, but there is no better definition.

The hugs, the kisses, the shared despair, these may ease her pain, but they do not erase the marks to her heart.

The disbelief, on her third birthday only four months after the separation, when her Dad showed up with the girlfriend's daughter in his arms, admonishing Gen and her little friends to be nice to her. A sweet, pretty little nymph the same age as Genevieve, who probably just wanted to go to a party…but didn't the man have one brain cell in his head?

In the event there is any doubt that a child of three can feel mortification, anger and humiliation, when Gen's father bent down to kiss her goodbye, she spat in his face…he was so shocked he slapped her, then hurried out the gate to his car.

I have nothing nice to say about myself either. After weeks of being alternately distraught and terrified at the depth of my daughter's misery, angry at what he was putting us through, I grabbed her and shouted after he left, "We have to be nice to him if we want him to come back, why did you do that?!" I screamed at my hurt little angel.

What misguided part of my brain thought she could show restraint, kindness and forgiveness, when I was so filled with anger myself I could easily have killed him with my bare hands. Gen was right… she would have suffered less if we had gotten him right out of our lives, right then.

By striving to accommodate his new life, by accepting the few bits and pieces of time he found for Genevieve, we spent years jumping every time the phone rang, pretending we weren't hoping the call was for her... only to have to witness the disappointment dull her beautiful eyes and shrivel her body… she would just fold into herself, and I could only offer such small comfort.

It was during these first months of hell, way before I learned that we make our own hells, one way or another, way before it became clear that my main concern should be to focus on *what are my goals, and how can I best achieve them,* rather than problems I was convinced others were causing me… it was right about here while I was floundering around in shock, that this was not a little *time out…* this was *goodbye;* that mother and son turfed me out of my buyer/manager position at Granny's up-market clothing boutique. My presence apparently not to the girlfriend's liking.

We were not divorced, they were not married, yet there I was, out on the street. It was a toss-up for me whether to curse the Watusi's greed and insecurities, or my husband's weakness.

PEARLS AND LACE UNDIES

As if I wasn't in a precarious enough financial position to incite the Gods of Wrath and Pathos, I walked away from the wreckage of our marriage without securing the house for Gen and myself.

Our beautiful beachfront house, the "Matrimonial Home" as Bahamian lawyers like to call it, the house that her Dad and I bought together a few months into our marriage. The house that by rights both moral and legal would provide shelter for mother and daughter… this house went to Dad.

The house we lived and loved in. The elegant new marble and glass house furnished at great expense by the New York couple who built it as their dream home, only to find six months later they were obliged to move back to the big city.

This very spectacular house had one huge bedroom overlooking the water, our own private secluded beach, his & her bathrooms, a fireplace in the living room, and ever changing views by day of turquoise and indigo waters as far as the eye could see. At night a string of fairylit townhouses curved around the beach in the distance at the far end of the bay. The house was perfect for the two of us.

The day after Genevieve's appearance into the world, my mind began designing a room just for her. A bigger house altogether in fact. Enclosing the upstairs patio would be easy, French windows all around and a raised 'tray ceiling' would make a perfect room for her. We would add an oceanview bathroom to die for, an Acqua Center for Gen and I overlooking the turquoise sea. A bathroom where even the Throne would have a glimpse of the view, and early morning ablutions would be sacred and serene, the face in the mirror reflected against the ever changing movement of the sea.

A magic room of ferns and mirrors, surrounding a step-up tub, forest green and extra large, snuggled against panoramic glass vistas. Luxuriating in bubbles in this secluded tropical corner, the coconut fronds and sky would meet the sea while one floated and dreamed.

A space of peace, of nature's greens and turquoises, a room I would enjoy as much as Gen would. In this designing mode, my mind soared on, adding a third bedroom that would be a a guest room overlooking the garden, plus a study and larger foyer on the ground floor under the newly created third bedroom… and in the garden, I would build the *piece de resistance*, a swimming pool with a semi-circular underwater bench built into the shallow end, providing seating for the round tile table… with a large, gaily colored umbrella in the center.

I envisioned the three of us sitting on that underwater bench one day soon, cool drinks on the table, a refuge from the heat of summer. A nice dream, but where would we get the money?

A year and a bit after Gen was born we leased the house to a genial banker and moved to one of Gen's Grandmother's properties where Gen would have her a room of her own. The house was old, not on the beach, but large and pleasant.

While the banker was paying a hefty monthly sum for our beachfront house, nicely paying off the mortgage and then some. I spoke to him one day of my plans for enlarging the house. He said he loved the idea, and didn't mind living in the house while the work was done around him… brave man.

And so I brought my dream house to life, with the help of a patient, talented young architect, the banker's rental money, and a small loan. The renovations took eight months, and the house was perfect; my dreams manifested right down to the umbrella and circular table in the pool.

We never moved back into that house as a family.

Which brings me to the lesson of 'be very careful what you wish for'. I wished for the house, dreamed and willed the house into being… did I perhaps forget to desire and pray and *see* the three of us living there, happy, healthy, and together?

* * * * *

Soon after Gen's dad and I split so unexpectedly, he said to me, "We need the banker to pay off the mortgage, so you and Gen can not live in the beach house". Numbly, I agreed. Nor, he said, could he afford the rent for the big house we were all living in together before the split. He was staying in the girlfriend's apartment, and insisted Gen and I move to a cheaper place.

I acquiesced for several reasons. In my befuddled state I thought, hoped, and prayed, that Gen might not miss her Dad so much in new surroundings; thought it might be better for her not to be in a house where she looked for her Dad in every corner, was reminded of him at every turn. Perhaps a change might be better for both of us. There was also the aspect of safety.

Alone with Gen now in the house, the large garden suddenly sprouted dark spooky corners at night. Break-ins were common in the neighborhood; dogs were being poisoned, and burglars prowled about at night blissfully aware of the inadequacies of the willing but underpaid, undermanned police force. Things I had not worried much about before now seemed frightening without a husband around; 'protection of the family' being one of the main mandates of a husband in my opinion.

I did not have a functioning brain to think things through, did not realize I had a choice. Had I dug in and stayed put, the finances would have resolved themselves between the rental income and our two salaries, extra security systems could have been added to the house Gen and I were in, and my great black dog, brought back with us from the first trip to France, could have lived inside instead of out, and been quite happy about the change.

Not having the right answers at the time, (indeed if there are any *right* answers), and being pressured by Gen's Dad to move immediately…he knew if I had time to think things through, we would have stayed put, I located a small two bedroom villa near the beach, a block from a small police station, thereby theoretically putting to rest my fears for our safety. Gen and I packed and moved in a daze. I do not remember her Dad being there, nor helping us with a thing. We were robbed within three months.

In broad daylight, while Gen and I were at the beach, romping in the surf with Boy, our big dog, pretending that all was well and life was good. Returning to the villa I found the sliding door wide open, the remains of my jewelry laid out meticulously on a pillow; a connoisseur taking his time, the good stuff gone forever, the fun fake stuff left as a remainder of the violation. The large diamond and sapphire ring given me by my mother, a gift to her from father in their romantic days, was still on my finger… where it remains to this day.

The danger that had narrowly missed us was more of a shock than the loss of the golden memories. Losing the jewelry was only another drop in this huge bucket of dramas we were swirling around in, trying valiantly to keep our heads above the muck. A few days later, a magical joke chose this moment to play itself on all of us, 'robber and robbee' alike.

A small pouch came to light in the final stages of unpacking. Abandoned in the last few months of our turbulent marriage, a silky bag of sexy lingerie with more than the usual secrets was tucked away in the bottom of a nondescript box. Jewelry, really good jewelry, long forgotten by me in the months of upheaval, was hiding shyly in the pretty lace underwear of my other dreams.

Cool white faces alive with light, here were the perfect pearls Gen's Dad gave me the day she was born, the one piece of jewelry I truly cherish. Camouflaged in a flowered negligee was the emerald and pearl bracelet given me by his mother as a peace offering on a day of relative calm. Silver Napoleon coins found by my brother when digging around in the attic of one of father's French farmhouses, rained out of a silken bag. Gold Kruger Rands from my days in South Africa winked merrily up at me from the softest lace undies. Mint gold coins from the King of Bhutan's coronation, a gift from the Tibetan monks…a kings ransom, a treasure refound. I sat down and cried with the joy of it.

Oh, the ups and downs of our life. The joy was fleeting. Gen's life turned from miserable to mean. The big house we recently left had a large pool, it was spacious, and attractively redecorated. A rather gloomy old house I had brightened with skylights and bay windows. A house that made others think we must be "Somebody."

We lost that status when Gen and I moved to the small rented villa. The move meant little to me, just one more unpleasant nuance to deal with. For Gen it was a disaster. The parents of her little friends decided we weren't good enough for them, or their kids. Bit by bit the kids became very "busy"; no time to visit Gen; no invitations forthcoming to visit. Ostracized.

Am I too harsh on these fickle parents? Was it perhaps nothing to do with our less worthy location…and more to do with my occasional rantings that put these parents off? Was I perhaps ranting all the time? I have no idea, I honestly don't know, can only guess, never had the courage to ask.

Gen and I went to the beach whenever we could. Making dribble castles in the sand cheered us both. Seeing who could turn the watery sand trickling between our fingers into the tallest curlicue tower made us laugh.

Gen seemed happy then… but I couldn't help thinking, was she really happy in this moment? Was I the only one thinking how much she loved swimming with her Dad, how she must be missing that? Was her heart aching like mine…remembering her Dad tossing her in the air every day after work, saying he loved her "more than anything!" Remembering how I loved watching her surprised face burst into laughter and joy midair.

Questions she was too little to answer, questions I dared not ask…unspoken questions answered by her tears every evening.

Now, years later, I am cursed with the conviction that leaving a familiar house makes it even harder for a child to deal with the separation of parents. Surely they would be better off in familiar surroundings, with only one huge change to deal with. Little friends visiting might not even notice dad was missing, fathers are often 'at work'. They might never be instilled with that subtle knowledge the move to a smaller house signaled to them through their parents, 'not only is this woman without a husband, her standing has now been drastically diminished'.

My belated advice to a mother with a small child finding herself faced with an unwanted divorce (with or without a second woman on the scene); "**Never give up the house!**" Sit tight and let him figure out how he is going to pay for His and Her residences.

Adding insult to injury, with much speed and little grace, Gen's Dad moved out of the girlfriend's apartment within a few short months of our move to the little villa …and installed his new brood in our beautiful beachfront house.

Was it possible that I lovingly put in all that time and effort… plus our combined incomes, into a house for his new girlfriend and her kids? Do you think the girlfriend would have held on to him with such vigor had the residences been reversed? My vote is no. However I can not fault her tenacity, only my stupidity. Still, I'm unable to let this go.

I don't blame this crafty woman entirely for taking over Gen's Dad, afterall I left him dangling out there for her to grab, I just can't forgive him for not making a stand to include his daughter in his new life.

Easing my guilt only very slightly over this dilemma is the fact that had we not moved to the villa, we were unlikely to meet the owner of the lovely house next door, a house that I was to purchase just a year later. Sometimes that makes me feel a bit better. That and the fact that we have managed to survive.

* * * * *

Gen started kindergarten in September at Lyford Cay School. She was not yet three. Although younger than all the kidlets in her class, I hoped being with other children would help her forget missing her Dad so much.

Lyford Cay is a private community at the Western tip of New Providence island and is famous for many things; mega-yachts, impossibly wealthy people, magnificent homes, a lush golf course, a Colonial club house complete with theatrical central staircase, and a dining room cleverly hiding a twenty foot section in the high vaulted ceiling that rolls back to reveal the stars on cool, clear nights. Impeccable lawns and tropical gardens surround a swimming pool unique only for the daily rental price of the adjacent cabanas, which open onto both the pool on one side, and the lawns leading to the sea on the other.

Lyford is all of this, yet one of its most attractive features is little known. Protected and hidden inside the guarded entrance to the community, is a little jewel of a school. Originally large enough for only a hundred or so children from kindergarten to grade six, the school was the grateful recipient of a financial infusion from an American businessman bringing a large portion of American wealth with him when he moved to the Bahamas. The newer buildings are beautiful, and the school is almost doubled in size.

Gen loved her school, was blissfully happy there and had a knack for learning everything quickly. I was thrilled she had something fun to do while I dealt with making a life for us.

Then suddenly a change… and not a good one.

Before Gen was four, her dad transferred his girlfriend's two children from government schools to Gen's school. Now there was nowhere to turn without bumping into reminders of her dad's defection, his betrayal, his new family. Genevieve wanted to be part of this new family, I wanted her to be part of it, but the girlfriend would have none of it. And now the two children were at Genevieve's school, wanting to be friends, but confused that their natural friendship with Gen was not allowed by their mother.

And it does not get better…a few months later Gen's dad and his girlfriend had their baby. The new little brother was joyously welcomed into their family, a mile down the road from our villa. Gen wanted to hold and coo over her little brother too, but rarely got to see him. The year after that, a sweet little baby girl brought the number of children in their house to four.

In the space of two years Gen's Dad went from having one child to five,…one of his, two of hers, and two of theirs. He had a great family for Gen to become a part of. She would no longer be an only child, something he had regretted about his own childhood.

But a happy family life with them was not in the cards for Genevieve. Married to Gen's Dad now, this stepmother wanted no reminders of her husband's first child, would tolerate her with them as little as possible.

There must have been good moments when they were together, but the overall memory of this part of Gen's life was one of being shut out, of watching helplessly as a happy family life evolved down the road without her.

Yet she couldn't get away from them either. Now we were tripping over the stepmother every morning and afternoon in the small school parking lot. Watching from my car one morning as she passed Gen with her two kids on their way to class, I actually saw this mean spirited woman refuse to say hello to my child, refuse to let her children hug Genevieve, yanking them away hurriedly, saying "She is NOT your sister," forcing them to ignore her shy smile and greeting… ruining Gen's morning, ruining her day at school, trying to ruin her life.

Genevieve began to feel miserable, unsure of herself and her place in life. A terrible change from her previously happy school demeanor. Gen's little schoolfriends noticed her gradual retreat from their play, noticed she sat by herself more and more instead of joining in… noticed something was altered… something that allowed them to tease her without fear of reprisal, something that made her an outsider where before she had been one of them. Six and scared, the sharks began circling.

My sweet girl began getting sick… stomach aches, sore throats, ear-aches, crying fits, headaches, temper tantrums and desperate attempts to get out of going to school… *afraid* to go to school… every day a trauma for both of us just to get her ready, both of us finding it increasingly difficult to enter the schoolgrounds where there was always a good chance of running into the Space Invader.

Sometimes Gen's Dad would drop the kids off to school. It is hard to know which was worse. She was thrilled to get a hug, but crushed to see him drive up with the two stepchildren, to see them taking her place, knowing they spent their days and weekends with him while she got just a few minutes once or twice a week when he dropped them off. Which was worse, to see him or not to see him?

Perhaps seeing him. After a visit to her Dad's house when she was about five, he dropped her outside our villa. He was never able to bring himself to come inside, never said hello to me if he could help it, choosing to stay in the car with the window rolled up, so I would have to tap on it if I wanted to converse with him. This time he shouted something about her causing trouble, and drove off.

I held her close as she came into the house with tears in her eyes and a red welt on her arm. Sobbing, she explained she had told the stepmother's first two children, the little girl her age and an older boy, *"He is my real father, not yours"*. It was a desperate bid to maintain something of her own in that house, the house Gen had come home to the day she was born. That beautiful beachfront house where I added an entirely new wing just for her, with her splendid bathtub that overlooked the sea, where her Dad was now living with these other people. Taken over by them.

The stepmother had slapped Genevieve and told her children a confusing lie; "He is not *her* father, he is *your* father", then sent Gen home sobbing.

Barely able to contain my rage, I sought to explain the difference between adoptive fathers, stepfathers, and *Biological* fathers… and that YES, her Dad was her real father.

"Oh good" she said with relief and a sudden glow to her little face, "he is my *Logical Father*."

It would do no good to say a word to her father, to him the woman could do no wrong. He would say I made it up, or I put words in Gen's mouth, although how he could ignore the welt on her little arm was always beyond me. Impossible to tell Gen she couldn't go over there again, she lived for those visits. The welt on her arm healed, but the slap to her heart did not.

Finances very soon become a precarious muddle after The Split. Gen's dad paid for our villa, but my only income was from an overflow of rent on Granny's house that Gen and I had recently vacated. I had found Granny another tenant when we vacated, negotiating a substantially higher sum for her than she was getting from us….could I have been *more* accommodating?! Gen's dad and I were still trying to work out the finances 'amicably," no lawyers yet haggling and postponing as they do best, but things were looking grim, grimmer and grimmest.

Out of the blue I was approached by a friend who not too subtly said, "Since you have split up with your husband you will probably be needing a job… how would you like to run a Submarine?"

Knowing less about submarines than just about anything else, but spurred by the creeping realization of a possibly imminent, desperate financial situation, I replied "Well I just might like to do that, what does it entail?"

"Oh nothing much" he replied, "You just have to run this business in Nassau for a friend of mine, he's in the States and not allowed back into the Bahamas. He owns the submarine, a restaurant and a Marina."

Living between the U.S. and the Bahamas for years, the owner had recently landed himself on the Bahamian 'Stop List'. Neither he nor his private plane were welcome, without hard to obtain special permission. Something to do with his plane being in the wrong place at the wrong time, with the wrong cargo.

Relegated to being an absentee landlord, unable to come into the country to visit his assets or collect his income at will, this friend assured him I would be able to handle the submarine business quite capably. I was not about to disappoint either one of them.

The Nautilus was docked in Nassau Harbor alongside the large waterfront Restaurant named, what else, Captain Nemo's. Ninety-two feet long, the submarine had been designed and built in the States for an early James Bond movie; the builders missed the deadline, and the Nautilus missed the movie.

Embarrassed and woebegone, she sat in the designer's backyard for a few years, until being discovered by the aforementioned adventurous American who lived in the Bahamas, and was at that point still very welcome to do so.

Converted into to a glass bottom excursion boat, and loudly painted in glorious shades of yellow, white and blue, The Nautilus was allegedly dropped into the Florida waters under the cover of night to avoid a quarter million dollar bond set by the U.S. Coast Guard in the event the as yet untested vessel went straight to the bottom of their harbor.

The gaily painted submarine sailed proudly from Florida to the Bahamas without the slightest problem, shocking a few passing boat Captains into thinking twice about having their next cup of rum.

When I came on the scene, The Nautilus had been happily plying its way up and down Nassau Harbor for years, to the delight of tourists and locals alike. At the initial meeting with the captain and first mate, sitting in the gazebo office at the end of the dock overlooking the water, I watched a cruise ship pull into the large docks built for them further down the harbor. It occurred to me that those huge floating cities were an untapped source of business.

Before talking to the heads of the cruise ship lines, the submarine crew and I spent hours tarting up the interior of The Nautilus, working nights and Sundays.

This floating fantasy seated fifty two passengers. A row of portholes on either side of the vessel gave a view above water, and glass windows on the floor in front of each row of seats provided the underwater viewing. The sub had thirteen rows of seats, four across, with two seats on either side of the central aisle. The viewing windows in the floor were made of one inch thick, bullet proof glass. I assumed the bulletproofing had to do with hull stress requirements, as I never saw an armed fish in all the trips I took.

A spiffy looking ship now after all our hard work. Fancy new uniforms for Captain and crew, Buttercup, the 'King of Limbo' was hired to liven up the slow return trip from the fantastic Sea Gardens… and we were ready to go after the cruise ship business.

Cruise Directors first, then the ship Captains, then Management in the Florida offices. I smiled and talked and persuaded, got them to visit the ship, take a free trip… showed them why this was an excursion their customers couldn't live without. Within a month the first cruise line was signed up, tickets for the Nautilus ride would be sold onboard the cruise ships. Disney Princess Lines; the Big Red ships as they were familiarly known. Customers and income doubled, my boss very pleased, and as I had cut a per passenger deal with him, I was now making big money.

Sounds too easy? How about the agony of having my first major meeting with the Miami cruise ship boss in Nassau going awry due to there being *two* red Disney ships in port at the same time… and either he, or me, waiting at the wrong ship.

The Nautilus' American owner had been allowed into Nassau that day for a visit to see how things were going. He was waiting with friends and lawyers at a table in the Restaurant, his restaurant, waiting for me to return from the meeting with good news and join them for lunch.

Having to tell this group of men that the meeting had gone amuck, was something I just couldn't face. Not to make excuses, but in my inner state of alternating fury, bitterness, sadness, guilt and depression over my daughter's fatherless plight, I found it desperately difficult to focus on anything as mundane as meetings and making a living, when my darling was suffering.

Driving back from the ships, my hand began turning the steering wheel of its own accord towards our little villa, my only desire to flee, to jump into bed and hide from the world.

Too many times during our marriage my husband had told me that an idea I mentioned to him was "the stupidest thing he had ever heard." Until a few days later when I'd overhear him making the idea his own and passing it on to a friend, at which time it became a good idea.... some women don't mind this, but it annoyed me to the core.

This conditioning no doubt had penetrated my being, making it almost impossible to stand up now and do what I knew was the right thing, to do what I *had* to do.

I listened to my heart, and ignored my lurching, very afraid body. I drove back to the Restaurant in a daze, rather like a zombie, not having a clue how I was going to handle this.

The car was parked, and I was walking slowly down the dock toward the Restaurant and certain doom, when Someone finally came to my rescue. A Plan was whispered in my ear, a subtle reward for my bravery. Straightening my back, faking breezy confidence, I strode over to the table, said hello to the five men, and announced very casually, "We missed this meeting, will have to do it next week, what's for lunch?" and sat down in the chair reserved for me.

Completely stunned for several seconds, my boss and the other men recovered quickly, ordered lunch, and began talking of other matters.

Accomplished career women seem to be born knowing that this bold and unconcerned approach, not unlike the stance often taken by men, works a treat in any situation. I however, had only this minute received the message, and just in time too. I made it through the next hour without anyone at the table ever knowing how close I was to just folding, dying maybe, at the thought of delivering the news of that botched meeting.

Nowhere in the same league of difficulty, but needing finesse nevertheless, was finding the most diplomatic way of telling the King of Limbo he would have to trim his show down a bit for the inside of the Nautilus cabin…That it was **not ok** *to set fire to the limbo stick in the middle of the submarine.*

Buttercup was the King of Limbo, a wiry Bahamian with a body so limber he was the envy of many a Yoga teacher. Precariously balancing his limbo stick across the center aisle of the submarine, just 8 inches above the ground, he would ask passengers on either side to hold it steady… while he lit the stick on fire.

Chanting "How low can he go," Buttercup's knees would pass first under the blazing stick, then his horizontal body, followed by the cowboy hat on his head.

He had done this insane feat many times in the restaurant, inevitably to gasps of amazement from the crowd, however when I saw him light the stick in the middle of a full submarine with only one exit at one end of the vessel, and no way out at the other, the liability aspect choked me.

Buttercup and I settled on a compromise…he could not light the stick on fire, he could however blow a huge ball of fire out of his mouth down the middle of the ship once all kids were safely settled next to their parents. He usually had to do this twice; somehow the quick little Japanese missed the shot with their cameras, and asked so nicely, "again, again, please!!" that Buttercup could not resist, even though it meant pouring a large cupful of alcohol into his mouth before lighting up. This little pastime was not something I mentioned to the insurance company.

One fine day the Captain called back to the office on the VHF radio in a mild state of panic, forty minutes after the Nautilus headed out for the day's underwater viewing with a full load of passengers. "Mrs. A., the engine has stopped and we are drifting backwards onto the rocks by Paradise Island, what do you want me to do?!"

Well obviously, I wanted him to get that engine started again.

This is not a call you want to receive at all, and particularly with a precious cargo of tourists onboard. Isn't the Captain supposed to figure this one out? Apparently not, it was up to me.

Getting on the VHF radio, I asked a friendly harbor ferry driver to take me out to the beleaguered submarine.

Pulling close alongside, I clambered up the slippery steep sides under the eyes of the bemused passengers, and once upright, announced to all that they would be getting a second boat ride today, at no extra charge! It was imperative I made it look like an adventure. It would only take one person to start moaning, and we would be out $1,000 in refunds.

These were lighthearted passengers, we offered free Rum Punches on all the trips. They had been out over Mahoney's Shipwreck, a spectacular viewing point in twenty feet of crystal water, and were buzzing with the excitement of it. The sand here was littered with large bits of wreckage from an old English tanker, blown to bits by dynamite years ago after it ran aground and could not be shifted. This was home to 300lb groupers and the occasional shark, and therefore a more exciting trip than the placid Sea Gardens, but it had its inherent dangers…large swells for one, and now the Nautilus was drifting quickly, too quickly, towards the beach and rocks.

Transferring all the passengers safely to the ferryboat amidst the heavy swells was a heart stopper for me, but the Captain and I had to make it seem like it was a lark to the casual observer. We waved goodbye effusively to the departing boatload of happy customers, the ferry captain made signs he would come by the office for his money later, and all seemed well, but it was too soon to breathe a sigh of relief.

The rocks were only a hundred yards away and the other boat called to tow us was nowhere in sight. Could this be the birth of a new Happy Hour drink, "Nautilus on the Rocks"?

With the Captain moaning that it would do no good to try starting the engine… yes, only one engine, a heretofore very reliable Cummins diesel… I *ordered* him to try it again. The roar of that engine coming miraculously to life was the greatest sound in the world. The relief that washed over me was something so tangible it should be bottled and sold.

DRUG BOATS AND THE DEA

After six months of running the Submarine efficiently and profitably, I began to notice from my dockside office that the Restaurant employees, as well as the customers, looked less than happy. I tried to ignore this by quietly skirting the mainly empty tables on my way to and from the office, until one of the chefs intercepted me one day and asked, "Why don't you take over the Restaurant Mrs. A, *why don't you just turn it around the way you have the Submarine business?*"

Intrigued and a bit flattered, I replied "Well thanks, but I don't know much about the restaurant business, and the owner hasn't discussed it with me." That was rectified a week later by a phone call from the U.S. owner, "How would you like to run the Restaurant?" My first Gemini reaction was that of a startled deer who could talk,

"No thanks!" I gasped, and dashed off into the forest.

Upon reflection over the next few days, it appeared that although everyone knew I had zero experience in the Restaurant business, they still seemed convinced I could do this… then why couldn't I? Faint messages somewhere in the back of my brain (woman's intuition? inner voice?) were warning me the submarine might soon be moved from the Bahamas to the U.S., where the owner could run it himself, thinking perhaps to make more money than the monthly checks I was sending him. Although it was a move that would make sense for him as he was sitting over there twiddling his thumbs, it would leave me with no job or income…therefore I reconsidered the restaurant carefully.

The Submarine was running smoothly now, and not knowing any better, I thought, "How difficult can running a restaurant be?!"

As anyone who has been even peripherally involved in running a restaurant can tell you, there is *no limit* to how difficult it can be. "Difficult" becomes a tame, inoffensive little word when faced with the variety of catastrophes one crashes into when striving to pull up a rundown restaurant by the boot straps; let alone a large one with an oversized staff of fifty and an absentee owner for over a year.

I was blissfully unaware that what I was about to embark upon was rather like having a baby, there is no way to know how bad it can be until it is too late to back out.

So I took on the management of Captain Nemo's Waterfront Restaurant and Marina, planning to work on the things I knew best, a delicious menu, warm atmosphere, and excellent service. The tough stuff, the unknown territory… staff payroll and scheduling, food and beverage inventory, I would leave in the hands of the previous manager for a few months and work along with her. That was the plan. Within a week that lovely lady decided she did not want to be second in command and walked off the job. I was now running a 200 seat restaurant, overstaffed with fifty employees, by myself.

Did I mention a 28 slip marina came with the restaurant?

What a peaceful, innocent looking little bit of protected water it appeared to be. Coming by boat from the direction of the Paradise Island bridge, you cruised past the restaurant and made a sharp left into the marina. Or you could dock in front of the restaurant to pick up a few beers and a lunch order before heading out to snorkel, sun, picnic, party, etc. on the nearby small islands.

Several of the slips in the marina were occupied by boats suspiciously dark, sleek and over-powered for weekend frolics to the nearby exquisite beaches, however I paid them little mind. I wondered vaguely why I didn't see these expensive boats being used very often, in fact I noticed very few of them seemed to go out at all in the daytime. They paid their rent on time however, usually in U.S. cash, and being busy with the Restaurant, the Submarine business, and a messy divorce etc, etc, I really didn't give the boats much thought.

I became quite friendly with several U.S. Drug Enforcement Agency officers seated often at the bar in the restaurant having a quiet drink. The American Embassy was only a few blocks away, and this was just a convenient place for them to hang out…I thought.

All became clear the night DEA helicopters swooped over the marina with lights blazing and megaphones shouting, "This is the Police, stay where you are! I repeat, this is the Police, Do Not Move!"

Despite this friendly bit of advice, there was a clattering of fast moving feet in the darkness on the other side of the marina. My DEA "customers" vanished in hot pursuit, racing after the bodies attached to the fast moving feet; and the mystery suddenly became very clear. My peaceful little marina was harboring several well known drug boats.

The boat owners who didn't end up in jail as a result of the bust, the remaining ones that were quite happily plying their trade under surveillance, (DEA watching and waiting to be led to the Big Fish), these were the gentlemen I had to ask, in the most diplomatic way, to move their boats elsewhere. They were always courteous and respectful to me, didn't really know how to deal with a woman running the show, a white one at that, but having noted the absolute fear they instilled in the waiters and bartenders when they came in to eat or drink, it was obvious I had to watch my step with them.

One evening however, one group stepped over my polite boundaries. Two fast, gray, evil looking thirty-six foot Cigarette boats blew into the marina just at sunset, and a bunch of rowdy men and women swarmed up the dock and into the bar. They began throwing hundred dollar bills around like confetti while they downed twenty shots of tequila in the space of two minutes. A few more rounds of shots, cash flying into the till, and normally I would have been thrilled to have such a busy bar.

As the liquor flowed, the language deteriorated. The F word is a favorite in the Bahamas in everyday language, often added to the words 'Yea man' to make up an entire conversation. I will never get used to it and have been known to stop people on the street and ask them to behave when their language is offensive… usually they are so stunned they apologize. I hate to think passing tourists and children assume these ill spoken loudmouths represent the Bahamas, so it would appear to be a matter of pride to me more than any moral judgment. Asking them, "Didn't you learn any other words in school?" also seemed to give them pause for thought.

I digress again. As the liquor flowed, the voices got louder until there could be no mistaking the portent of the conversation. Pushing and shoving then ensued, all this in the space of fifteen minutes. The restaurant customers began looking uneasy, and I decided it was time for the bar customers to leave.

Despite my quiet signal to the bartender to stop serving the group, he continued to plunk down the shots. The rowdy group continued to guzzle everything he put before them. A slow burn heated up my insides and I sprang into action.

"Out! All of you out" I shouted loudly to anyone who would listen, jumping into the middle of the melee. I heard a couple of rude remarks about the "white woman not wanting their business" and a lot of muttering and grumbling. I grabbed the apparent leader of the group and said, "Your friends are not behaving properly, they're making the other customers nervous, I would like you to remove them."

"OK," he replied after a short but noticeable pause, then polite as can be, "I understand, sorry about the noise." And to his cohorts, "Come on guys let's move on." They clambered back onto their boats, gunned the five hundred horsepower engines, two per boat, and roared out of the marina, waving and cheering. I rounded on the bartender.

"Why didn't you stop serving them when I asked you to!?" The nicest guy in the world, and one of my best employees, Greg looked at me and said "Mrs. A, you don't have any idea who that was, do you?" It appears I had just rousted one of Nassau's biggest drug lords… out of jail on half million dollars bail, after allegedly murdering a policeman.

*****

This was a period of total chaos in our lives, Genevieve's and mine. Her dad and I were deadlocked with lawyers; any conversation between us was loud and furious, seething with frustration and anger. On the work front, the first records I obtained confirmed the Restaurant had been teetering on the brink of bankruptcy before I took it over; the fifty employees I inherited expected me to miraculously bring the place back to life and assure them their livelihoods… when I could barely assure my own.

As near as I could tell from a preliminary calculation of customers versus staff and jobs to be done, the business was overstaffed by at least fifteen persons, yet it was impossible to fire anyone unless they were in breach of one of the two basic rules set out by the labor board; no theft, and no fighting on the premises.

Catching someone stealing only caused another dilemma for me. When a woman employee with four kids at home is caught walking off with a large bag of our specialty "Johnny Cake' bread, my first reaction is to think, "she needs it"… and I haven't the heart to take it from her, let alone fire her.

This is a tricky place to be, to let her keep the bread while I still maintain some respect. In this case I opted for a deal. She would stay an extra hour the next day with no pay, making more Johnny Cake for the Restaurant. I was happy with that, and she was thrilled not to be fired. While I can not say it stopped food from walking out the back door, at least the losses were not so blatant thereafter.

Sullenness, unwillingness to adapt to new policies, that was the name of the game in the beginning. I would say to a different person every day, "No, we do not walk over napkins laying on the floor of the dining room, we pick them up… we do not tie up the reservation line for hours chatting with friends… we do not have friends drop by for free food and drink". These were not fireable infractions, merely daily occurrences.

Having staff meetings was not the answer, there would only be a line of blank faces and no sign of feedback. To find what would motivate these people, to see them happy to work heart and soul with me, was not a simple thing.

The key it turned out, was singling out two smart women who could also see the possibilities of making the place a success, then earning their trust by asking opinions and giving them responsibility. They soon began recruiting their own team, people they could count on to get the job done, and suddenly everyone wanted to be on a team. It was magic, and a beginning, but I was already a wreck.

Running the submarine business, working at the restaurant til all hours, worrying about my sad little kidlet at home with a babysitter when she needed me, worrying about the weekly five figure payroll, worrying about the lawyers, worrying about what a wreck I'd made of my life…all of this banging around in my head without respite.

Is it any wonder I had an attack of some sort? Had to call the ex, who rushed me to the emergency room hyperventilating and palpitating (me, not him).

I was topped up intravenously with gallons of fluids and told to "*rest*." Such a useless bit of advice, don't those doctors think we would rest if we could?

On top of all this, things got worse if possible between us all, the stepmom, Gen, her Dad, and me. I had qualms about letting Gen go to her Dad's when he invited her to spend the night with them, knowing the stepmother could not tolerate her… or more likely it was the reminder of me she could not tolerate.

What if there was a fire, or an accident? This woman certainly would not be worrying about rescuing my little pumpkin, she had four of her own to worry about.

I didn't have the heart though, to tell Gen she couldn't visit her Dad's house. She lived for being asked to spend the night with them, wanted more than anything to be part of a real family. This was not a time to tell either of us that "real families" can be made up of any number of people, even two. Every time she was invited she would put all the troubles behind her and go to their house with enthusiasm and a light heart…but some trauma would invariably occur to ruin her happiness.

Somewhere in here there was an unspeakable incident, Gen being chased around the house by the older stepbrother with a kitchen knife, where once again she was somehow to blame and sent home in tears… details best forgotten.

Crushing blows to her heart, too much for her little spirit. When finally neither of us could take anymore, I transferred Gen to another school at the other end of the island. It was too little too late. A January semester, not the start of a new year. A hard time to fit into a bigger school. The headaches escalated, not just during the week, but now weekends as well.

Weekends when she should have been outside playing or swimming, at the beach, or off with friends, Gen was in a dark room with an ice pack on her head. By the time she was ten we had seen every doctor on the island. Two cat scans confirmed there were no physical abnormalities, the headaches most likely caused by emotional stress. We were even told by an Indian doctor at the Government Hospital that, *"If she has had the headaches for three years and is still alive, it can't be too serious."* Was it just me, or shouldn't a diagnosis like that be awarded with a smack to the head?

Throughout this entire time Gen still managed to get top grades, though regularly missing one or two days of school a week. Headaches, Bronchitis, Strep throat, one after another. Absent from school for doctor's visits, drowsy from antibiotics, tons of schoolwork to make up, still she slogged on. As one teacher put it in grade seven, "If she were able to attend school every day, she would be in college by now."

Lost wretched years…the agony of that first Christmas without her dad when Gen was not quite three, pretending to have a cheerful two-person Christmas. Watching my little angel stretching up to place ornaments on the tree, alone. Shaking my head to dislodge visions of her Dad's new kids a mile down the road romping around their huge tree together, with two loving parents overseeing the friendly chaos.

Buying Christmas presents to put under the tree from Santa to myself was a Yuletide chore that took exceptional fortitude, as did wrapping the joyless gifts just to have boxes to open along with Gen's presents; her delight at watching me open them as great as when opening her own.

Years of anguish, Gen's and mine, when the stepmom would not make Gen feel welcome in her Dad's house, did not want her to be part of their family, would rarely let the new little brother and sister come and play with Genevieve at our house even though they asked to do so repeatedly. Worst of all, admitting the real wretch was not so much the wicked stepmother as the father, who sanctioned such meanness.

It was too much, I was going crazy dealing with the guilt of ruining my daughter's childhood, the stress of overworking myself at the restaurant from eleven a.m. often until two a.m. doing the accounts,,,which become a blur of undistinguishable figures at that hour, and making myself sick with worry that Genevieve was stuck at home with a housekeeper and no mom.

By the time she was eight, Gen knew the business well, and would call to ask me to come home at 9pm instead of midnight or later. If I replied that I couldn't, she would say, "How many customers do you have Mom?' I'd look around and make a quick guess, then she would ask how many waiters were working. After hearing the number she made a quick calculation and said, "They can handle it Mom, come on home." How do you say no to that logic?

The time after school between the hours of four and six p.m. when I would dash home to be with her, was only an exercise in frustration as I fought to stay awake enough to play with her. Ongoing negotiations with her Dad and lawyers for some kind of a settlement were sapping any energy I had, and dragging myself out of bed to get Gen ready for school in the morning was a tremendous ordeal. In the midst of this, the worst time of my life, something caught my eye on the front cover of a People Magazine at the supermarket. Inside was an article that saved me.

It was written by a lovely old doctor in California, complete with an old sepia photo of a woman so exhausted, so frazzled and lost, it could only have been taken in an asylum. I sent him a nice photo of Gen and I together, and wrote that, "While I looked fairly attractive on the outside, his photo of the unknown, indescribably miserable lady, was me to a T on the inside."

He replied with a thoughtful letter and recommendations regarding long-term postnatal depression, and advised me to go easier on myself. To accept that I had too much to cope with for one person to bear easily, let alone expect to be cheerful about it.

And that's all it took…hearing that someone was finally listening and trying to help, that in itself was enough to give me such huge relief.

A relief to be able to let my guard down, to finally understand that in the midst of the fast moving chaos that was my life during and after the split of our tiny family, I could not continue to blame myself for the things I thought I should have done, or should be doing differently.

While the gentle California doctor could not prescribe medications given the distance between us and not seeing me personally, the knowledge that I was doing as well as could be expected under the circumstances, and his caring enough to write a long helpful letter… that was enough to put me on the road to physical and mental recovery.

Still, I was very tired. I took Gen to and from school every day until she was eight, when she began to take the bus. After dropping her off in the morning, I would often stop on the side of the road and nod off for ten minutes, before hitting the road again. Tired as I was, picking her up in the afternoon was always a pleasure, and seeing that great smile when she saw our car and came running, that made everything worthwhile.

One day on the way home from school, when Gen was about six, she said out of the blue in her casual, sweet way, referring to her stepmother,

"Mummy why is she so *brown*!? Her hair is brown, her eyes are brown, her face is brown, even her feet are brown, why is she so brown!?"

As the Bahamas is predominantly a black country, I was intrigued to hear this was the first time she had noticed any difference in skin color. I replied thoughtfully, "Well Pumpkin, there are lots of different colors of skin in the world, that's what makes it fun."

"Well," she said, running her little hand over my lightly tanned arm, "your skin is so soft and pretty Mum, your skin is *Honey English*."

I could not know, that sweet day when her words brought a mist to my eyes, that she had given me more than a memory. Genevieve had given me the title of the book I had not yet begun to write.

* * * * *

THE SAUDI PRINCE

Delving into unpaid Restaurant bills the first couple of months after taking it over, it became apparent that over a quarter million dollars was owed to banks and food and beverage suppliers; several of whom were not interested in delivering anything until past bills were paid. As there are only three or four food suppliers in Nassau, and the restaurant owed every one of them money… lots of money… I had to work out something quickly.

Giving this unwelcome but not entirely surprising news to the owner during a meeting in Miami, he threw his hands in the air and said, "You are on your own, I'm not putting another penny into that place!" He signed his shares in the company over to me for one dollar.

I did not execute the documents to transfer the Company to my name for fear of becoming liable for the debts, and continued to run the business in whatever capacity that move entailed.

Single-handedly, I struggled with this drowning monster, and I specify *single-handedly* for the dozens of people who said at one time or another, "Oh Honey, are you running this place for your husband?" or even more annoying, "Did you get the Restaurant in the divorce?"

With no money available for improvements, magic had to be performed in the dining room with paint and plants. The menu was revitalized. Tasty 'broiled lobster' replaced boiled, Grilled Grouper was now on the menu as well as our famous Smudder, steamed grouper smothered in onions and tomatoes. We had 'Peas n Rice' to die for, and the best *Johnny Cake* in town.

The changes thrilled most of the staff, and they soon learned a happy customer is one who tips well. The weekend band turned the place into a hot spot… customers dancing in the entrance and up and down the dock, with the irrepressible Bahama Mama waitresses "shaking their booty" to and fro between kitchen and tables.

The Nassau taxi drivers, a club all unto their own, joined our team. They soon discovered that when customers asked where the best seafood was, if they recommended our Restaurant, dropped them off and picked them up after lunch or dinner, they were sure to be rewarded with much thanks and extra tips. We installed a shady shelter at the gate for the waiting drivers, and always made them welcome on the premises, which they appreciated.

So much so apparently, that customers sometimes asked if I owned the Taxi company. They said no matter which Taxi they had asked during their stay in Nassau about the best place for seafood, the answer was always the same, "Captain Nemo's". This upswing in word of mouth on the Restaurant was the most important change in our fortunes that I remember, and the taxi drivers are to be thanked.

To this day I can climb into a taxi in Nassau, and stand a good chance of the driver remembering me, or arrive at the airport to have a smiling face step out of the crowd to shake hands, or I'll hear a yell with a friendly wave, "Mrs. A, Hello!". It makes Nassau almost bearable.

The Restaurant was taking shape. Tricky staff scheduling was conquered, staff numbers were trimmed from 50 to a more efficient 36. Luckily the ones I was least sad to see go were also the ones most likely to breach the 'no fighting, no stealing rules'.

Sunglasses of one employee were lost, then found on the face of a co-worker, and the ensuing battle removed two troublemakers. Domestic disputes between staff having off-work relationships were settled by plate throwing episodes in the kitchen, or knife threats between the grill and the steam table…frequent events in the beginning that made my life easier in the long run, culminating in one or two less people on the payroll each time.

Food purchasing from the recalcitrant suppliers was even running smoothly, a satisfactory deal having been made to pay them C.O.D., plus paying a bit extra towards the old bills.

One thing still missing was a system to track daily sales. Without the benefit of a computer in the beginning and no previous records available, the first month of manual tracking in a ledger gave me a shock. We were taking in over one hundred thousand dollars a month…I was running a million dollar business!

I had to sit down and absorb that. Over $100,000 coming in per month, but the same amount or more going out. The trick was to capture some of it.

During the months it took to learn how to wrest profit from the lean margins, unforgettable stories came out of this restaurant business, some amusing, some not so amusing. This first one is merely amazing…

One lovely sunny afternoon we arranged several waterfront tables with extra care, to accommodate fifteen very VIP guests for a three p.m. luncheon, a Saudi Prince and his family. The Manager of their hotel called to ask that I be there personally to assure all went smoothly.

At exactly three p.m. the Prince and his entourage flowed down the dock and into the Restaurant dressed in a mix of Western wear and traditional Eastern garb.

Once they were seated and ordering refreshments, I offered their Bahamian driver a drink. Recognizing him from my submarine days as a bit of a pirate, I was not surprised when he asked for a tip for recommending the restaurant to the group.

"Stanley" I said patiently, "these people have had reservations for two days, look at the tables all ready for them," and I pointed in the direction of the happy group. Puzzled but stubborn, he replied that they *couldn't* have had reservations… he had been driving them all day and he had just stopped by when they got hungry.

Suddenly all became clear… too clear. Striding down the dock was a *second* wave of fifteen Saudis, obviously the ones we had prepared the tables for.

Looking at the fifteen enjoying themselves in the best waterfront corner, flowers and silverware in chaotic disarray, I said to myself in disbelief, "Who are these people?!"

The first Prince was in fact a cousin of the second. They greeted each other effusively, as surprised to find themselves in the same place at the same time as I was. Please tell me what are the chances of two Saudi Princes, each with an entourage of fourteen, arriving at the same Restaurant within ten minutes of each other, at three in the afternoon.

My wonderful dining room staff sprang into action, the kitchen went into overdrive… everyone it seemed, wanted the Grilled Lobster the restaurant was famous for, and thanks to the graciousness of the Prince whose tables had been usurped, all went exceedingly well. Stanley the taxi driver got his tip and my apologies.

The dining room was the fun part of the business. Chatting with happy customers, meeting people from every corner of the world, this was the easy part. Holidays however, could abruptly become a nightmare. On one or two nights of the year the other excellent seafood restaurant in town, The Poop Deck... a legitimate nautical term I believe, closed on either Christmas or Easter, *the* busiest times of the year. At Captain Nemo's we could be sure of one thing, that we would be swamped. We were careful to check dates with them beforehand and put on extra staff, but even then things can go wrong, isn't there something about 'the best laid plans of mice and men?'

Our number one hostess could not be scheduled this particular evening. Keeping the fifty or so tables and two hundred people revolving smoothly when we were busy was a trick she managed perfectly. She was firm with bullying guests who insisted they had reservations but didn't, gracious with guests who might have to wait twenty minutes for a table, careful to keep the waitlist names in the correct order... I on the other hand dreaded that part of the business.

Our number two hostess was charming but did not have the same mastery of the dining room as my favorite lady. Trouble started early on this evening, with guests showing up saying they had been told when calling for reservations, "It isn't necessary, just come on down!"

The cashier/receptionist swore she'd never told anyone to, "Come on down," but I wouldn't put it past her if she didn't feel like writing all those names down.

By eight o'clock there was a line of forty people backed up on the dock. Taxis were dropping couples at the gate, purposely scooting out without giving the security guard a chance to explain there would be a long wait, leaving guests stranded at our place, and desperate for a meal.

Of course our intercom system was not working that night, and by the time I thought to send someone to the gate to tell security to turn the taxis away it was too late. Fifty yards up the dock from the restaurant, the guard hadn't paid attention to the pile up, although I wonder where he thought we were stashing all those bodies he was letting in.

The bar, the dock, the outside patio and the entrance by the band were swamped with hungry couples. My hostess number two, lovely Loranda, looked up at the mass of faces, looked at me, and said weakly, "Mrs. A, I don't feel well"… and fainted on the spot.

With help from the crowd, we picked her up and casually leaned her against a post for support while I signaled to a passing waiter to help her out of the dining room. At that point I went on remote pilot… don't remember what I did or how we served everyone.

I do remember seeing my great friends from Westport Massachusetts at the bar having a drink. They lived across the harbor on a large yacht in Hurricane Hole and Gen and I had great times sailing with them on my rare days off. Tonight they jumped in to help bus tables and take orders. It was total chaos, but with their help we made it through the night and lived to laugh about it.

Another evening's traumatic events you may or may not find amusing, depending on how dark your sense of humor is.

New Years Eve, with only fifteen minutes to go before popping champagne for two hundred Swedish guests who had booked the entire restaurant. Lobster dinners had long been devoured, the fire breathing limbo dancers exhausted, the band valiantly keeping everything lively with a soft mellow tempo. Suddenly Charlie, a tall, and heretofore pleasant busboy, chose the moment to take offense at something said to him by one of our slightly inebriated marina tenants sitting at the bar. Going apparently berserk on the spot, he chased the man up and down the dock with a large knife he wrestled from the head chef on a dash through the kitchen.

Somewhere mid-chase the sound of a breaking bottle zinged back to me from halfway up the dock; a bottle obviously being smashed against a piling to create a better weapon.

While I calmly dialed the police in a show of having things totally under control, my mind was well aware that this could end badly; the police would be too late… if they showed up at all. This did not auger well for the New Year.

Loyal waitresses, chefs and the bartender saved the night by jumping on Charlie's back and riding him up the rest of the dock, out through the security gate and into the arms of the burly guard before any real damage was done. In his office at the end of the dock, busy greeting guests and directing taxis, the security guard hadn't heard the ruckus. He now held Charlie in a headlock, awaiting instructions.

Dealing with the police, assuming they chose to appear eventually, would interfere with the New Year Countdown…right now I had champagne to serve.

The boat owner was unharmed, a fast runner for his drunken state, but clamoring for me to put Charlie in jail. As the only wound was to his pride, and it was now five minutes to midnight, I made an executive decision. I asked him to return to the restaurant and ring in the New Year with us.

To the now submissive Charlie I said, "Don't let me catch you near this property again." The guard held him immobile.

"Yes Boss Lady" he replied politely, calmed down and ashamed. I instructed security to let him go, and Charlie took off like a tall rabbit.

When I saw him on the street a few weeks later, he apologized and had the nerve to ask for his job back. We both had a good laugh as I said, "Charlie, you've got to be kidding, you're lucky you are not in jail!"

"Yes Boss Lady, you're right. Thanks and I'm sorry."

Since Gen was six or seven, she had been coming to the restaurant with me a few nights every week. She loved to help, checking tables with me, chatting with the customers, or doing homework in my office…often falling asleep in the huge overstuffed chair I bought for that purpose.

We had very little time together otherwise, and my heart was always torn leaving her at home with housekeepers, so while this was not an ideal way to be together, it had been better than nothing.

Gen was luckily tucked up in bed at home that crazy night, however there was no getting around it, the Restaurant was not a safe place for her to be. Now we would have even less time together…I had to get out of this business.

OF KIDNAPPERS AND LIMES

Selling the restaurant was not so much a choice as a necessity. I had been handling every aspect of the operation myself for six years. Although I had several wonderful people working with me, I needed a partner, someone to share the decisions and responsibilities, as well as the profits. I could not run it by myself any longer, but the three-year lease I had just been granted was not long enough to entice a good partner, and what sort of partner would I have made? I was burned out.

It was not so much the operation of the business that finally got me down, it was the Union. As soon as the restaurant began to turn around and become successful, I was dragged into a three year battle with the local Hotel and Caterers Union for trumped up claims against the previous owner, to the tune of $100,000… for Christmas turkeys and uniforms that past employees allegedly had not received, employees whose names the union was unable to supply.

The union was displeased with me. This is a bit of British understatement. From fairly early on in my tenure, in fact probably right from the night my least favorite waitress asked me to please talk to her husband for a minute, outside the restaurant. Assuming it was restaurant business, I stepped out onto the dock with her, only to be faced with a drunken and agitated slob heaving a baseball bat. It was 10pm and dark out on the dock, the security guard nowhere in sight.

I don't remember the husband's grievance, something to do with his wife having an affair with one of my cooks, which he wanted me to confirm. I wasn't sure if the bat waving erratically was for me or the cook, but ignoring him completely I said quite calmly to her, "You should not have brought this man here to talk to me in this state, you are endangering me and the customers, you are fired".

He swore then, and shouted that I could not fire her. My icy reply was worthy of a Clint Eastwood movie; "Watch me" I said and walked quickly back to the relative safety of the restaurant, called security on the intercom that was working this time, and had them both escorted off the premises.

And fire her I did. It turned out she was the union's Shop Steward, and while at the time I had no idea what a shop steward was, having never opened the thick copy of the union contract lying on the floor of my office, it soon became apparent from the union's frantic protests, that Shop Stewards are basically 'unfireable' employees.

The local Labor Board accepted my position that, "I would close the restaurant before taking her back." They overruled the union in my favor, and allowed the termination of the waitress. They asked the union to come up with a reasonable figure for her termination pay. The union officials negotiated fiercely with me, and in their anger made a slip in their math and ended up settling for $1,500 less than I had been prepared to pay. Thus began the union's vendetta against me.

I refused to read the union contract for the first year, a document signed by the absentee American owner months before I came onboard. Union officials repeatedly stopped by my office to quote a one liner buried somewhere in the contract stating, "Any new owner is bound by this contract."

To be bound by a contract I had never even read, let alone signed, was an affront to my common sense. Nor did I consider myself an owner in the legal sense, having never completed the necessary paperwork due to the possible financial liability issues.

So the battle started, interminable meetings called by the Union and their attorneys every month or so. At which I would repeat in alternating terms of politeness or anger;

"There is no way I will turn over a penny to these parasites, I *will* close the restaurant first…do they want to put 40 people out of work?

Or I would inquire; "Who is there to help the employees get their kids into the hospital on weekends when they need emergency treatment? I am. Who kept them all on the payroll using the last of my personal savings throughout the Gulf War, when there wasn't an American tourist to be seen on the island for weeks? I did.

And finally; "What did the union do for the employees except collect the same weekly dues whether they worked five days or two?"

The union officials were unable to answer these questions, although my logic was not lost on them, and it did not endear me to them. Their interminable "arbitration" meetings usually went on for hours. Five, six, sometimes seven hostile Bahamian men, union officers and lawyers, against one tired British lady. The numbers varied, but their ruthless assault did not.

I did have a lawyer accompany me to the first meeting. It became immediately apparent that it was a waste of money; no law firm wanted to bang heads with the Union. So there I sat alone, meeting after meeting, hour after hour, one against many... down but not out.

After a few months of these futile forced get togethers, my employees reported hearing scarcely veiled threats to kidnap my daughter from the restaurant; I began receiving late night phone calls to my house warning I was going to be shot; union officials would sit at the bar and harass the employees, sneering at them for working for "the white lady".

All of this and more I endured, I know not how. No help from the police who advised, "We are unable to set up phone taps, the phone company is not in possession of the appropriate equipment".

Dozens of wasted hours spent going to meetings that were canceled an hour after I arrived, due to no-shows on the other side. Worse hours endured when the meetings did take place, and came alive in the most negative of atmospheres. My enthusiasm for running the business was being crippled, all strength and creativity sapped.

The details of the reverse racism and insults I had to endure at the hands of the union officials and their lawyers will remain in my own private memory, locked in the bottom drawer of that elegant gembox box in my mind.

The months of hopeless wrangling over the monies they were claiming stretched into three years. Then finally the meeting came when it was obvious I was going to be the loser in this battle. Top on the agenda of the supposedly unbiased 'Chairperson' was not justice for the employer, but for the union; and the question now was not if I would have to pay... but how much.

Sensing a defeat that would put us out of business, I lost it. I insulted the lawyers, I insulted the union officials, I insulted the Chairperson. She smacked her hand on the desk and cited me for 'Contempt of Court'. That was it, there was no stopping me, I jumped up and shouted,

"Fine, just tell me what that means in this kangaroo court! Do I go to jail? Do I get fined? What exactly does 'contempt of court' mean here?!" In the deafening silence that ensued, it was obvious that no one had an answer.

I picked up my briefcase, and walked unchallenged out the door.

A week later there was a miracle. After three years of this fierce battle, out of the blue one morning on the front page of the local newspaper was a headline shouting what had been my silent scream for months… 'Union arbitration meetings a farce, unconstitutional, a kangaroo court'…and today *abolished*.

The union could no longer force employers into interminable meetings for the sole purpose of tormenting them and flaunting their power; now they could only *invite* them to a meeting. A well known attorney, nicknamed "Brave", had gone to bat for a besieged hotel owner in Freeport. He took the case all the way to the Supreme Court for a win.

Shortly thereafter a notice arrived in the mail politely inquiring if I would like to attend an arbitration meeting regarding the ongoing case, scheduled three weeks from date of notice. Just as politely I ticked the box marked NO, and mailed the notice back as requested. A month later I was advised by mail the case had been dismissed. Just like that.

But it was too little too late. Even the relief and rejoicing could not pull me out of my slump. The effort it took for me to function on a daily basis was enormous. I still had adrenaline enough to take care of the odd crisis, but the mundane weekly review of sales and purchasing figures just could not keep my attention.

The night security guards worried that I stayed til three a.m., then drove home alone on dangerous roads. I could not get the work done any other time, but at night the numbers blurred in front of my eyes. The figures would be a jumble, or move to an altogether different location on the page.

The good days when I could accomplish in half an hour what it would take others two hours to do were no longer. I was not running the restaurant any longer, it was running me…but how could I leave it? The place was my livelihood, and I had turned it into quite a good one.

After the first turnaround year, and excluding the timeout for the Gulf war when many businesses folded, never to recover, the restaurant served close to fifty-two thousand people a year. A thousand faces, lunch and dinner seven days a week, fifty-two weeks a year. I had to do the math one day when the FBI asked me to identify photos for an upcoming trial. Photos of a man whose alibi was, "lunch at Captain Nemo's and a chat with the owner," yours truly.

We had apparently discussed the Captain's cocktail party I attended the night before on the U.S. Navy boat docked a few hundred yards from the restaurant. I could not understand why I remembered the party onboard the Navy vessel, and not the man in the photo...a large man wearing a t-shirt with a huge shark emblazoned on his chest... was I losing my mind?

The FBI agent asked how many people we served a year. When I gave him the figures and we worked out the total, he laughed and said there was no way I should be able to remember that particular man. He was impressed however when we dug up the lunch check with the exact items that the large man swore he had consumed. I was mystified that he would remember exactly what he ate and drank, unless he *planned* to use the restaurant and lunch as an alibi if caught at whatever he was up to at the time.

I didn't hear the conclusion of the case, but would have been interested to know whether the retrieved lunch tab was Sharkman's ticket to freedom.

There were many days when the Restaurant was a wonderful place to be. People from different countries came year after year to see us again, to tell us what an important part of their vacation the Restaurant had been. One couple from Italy returned four nights in the same week, hopped off to Vegas to get married, then came back to see us for one last dinner before heading back to Europe.

Sell? Don't sell? What was the business worth? I didn't own the buildings, had only a three-year lease, but a great European and American customer base.

"Yes, I have to sell, I can't do this any longer". Six years overseeing forty employees by myself seven days a week, with a little daughter at home who was managing the best she could within the chaos that was our lives... how much damage was being done? That was the overriding question always in my mind.

At what point exactly it all became too much to bear, I don't know. I do know the time came when I couldn't face dragging myself to the restaurant one more day, one more night…I was tired, I was blurry, I was gone.

The final decision to let it all go came down to a lime. The day, or rather the night of reckoning came two days before my seventh Christmas in the restaurant business. Any type of holiday in Nassau means the food and beverage suppliers can close for days at a time… but the restaurants stay open.

Therefore a certain amount of planning is required. Nothing strenuous, just *thorough* planning, as everything that might be needed over the Christmas holiday has to be ordered ahead of time. Friday at six p.m. all suppliers except the supermarkets would close until the next Tuesday morning.

Friday afternoon I double checked everything with the purchasing office.

"Did we get everything the Head Chef ordered?"

"Yes".

"Are you sure we have everything we need to go for three days, lunch and dinner?"

"Yes, yes, and yes."

From home early Friday evening I called the Restaurant and spoke to the cashier. "I am on my way, making a last stop at the supermarket before it closes, does ANYBODY need ANYTHING!?"

"No, we are all set" they said.

I zipped around our local Winn Dixie supermarket grabbing last minute items for the house. As I passed the fruit counter a huge box of bright green limes caught my eye. I thought how pretty they were, and dashed on.

Arriving at the Restaurant at 7:30pm I did a quick dining room check and saw everything humming smoothly. After an hour of paperwork in my office I went through the dining room again, chatted at a few tables, checked with the hostess that couples waiting happily at the bar would soon have a table, and headed back to my office via the outside terrace.

I didn't make it.

As I passed a table of four, one of the gentlemen said, "Excuse me, could I have a piece of lemon to go with my lobster?"

"Of course, I'll get you one," I said, and glanced at his plate. Something that resembled a quarter of a grapefruit was hulking over the beautifully grilled lobster.

Pushing through the double swinging doors to our large kitchen where the flurry of activity was purposeful and competent… three of our six chefs working tonight, two dishwashers going at top speed and an assortment of waitresses picking up orders on huge trays I would never get the knack of balancing, I had a moment of pride.

How smoothly things were running. The chef I'd recently hired at great expense to organize the kitchen…rather than overseeing everything from fritters to freezers myself, was working well, and life seemed good; all except for that damn lobster plate without a lime or lemon. We used local limes instead of imported lemons whenever possible.

"Derek," I said to the head chef, busy doing something fancy and decorative with bright red tomatoes, "would you hand me a lime please." Derek reached into a box by his side and passed me something large, greenish-white, and suspiciously like a grapefruit; it did not even look like a 'sour', the native bitter orange that is delicious when making conch salad, but does not pass for either a lime or lemon in anyone's book.

I studied the oversized, thick skinned, dried up object in my hand. It was definitely related to the strange object on the customer's plate in the dining room.

Still with hope in my heart I said, "No, this won't do, where are the limes?"

Derek didn't bother to look up from his project, just waved aimlessly in the air and said, *"That's what I met when I reached."* Translation: "When I got here for my shift at 2pm this afternoon, that's what had been delivered instead of limes."

Quite calmly, given the rush starting inside me, I said,

"I just came from the supermarket, there were bushels of limes, why didn't someone let me know?"

He shrugged his shoulders dismissively. I bit my tongue. Silently, deftly, I cut a small slice of the strange fruit so it might conceivably pass for a pale, juiceless lime, and took it to the customer.

After graciously setting the little plate next to him with the blighted offering, I walked out of the restaurant and up the length of the dock, seeing nothing, hearing nothing, muttering under my breath, "That's it, I will not be sabotaged again by this sloppy, 'don't give a damn' attitude. We have been doing this for over six years, we should be able to get it right by now. I put my life's blood into this place and no one else gives a damn. This is just too much - that's it, I am selling this place."

On and on I ranted. Steam must have been coming out of my ears because our lovely security guard, the young man who was desperate for a good job two years ago when his fiancée became pregnant, stopped me mid-stride and said, "Mrs. A, are you alright?"

"No, I am not alright Johnny, I am not alright at all. I am mad, I am angry, I am frustrated, and I am too tired to do this anymore. I am selling the place tomorrow".

At the stricken look on his face I felt a terrible pang, but repeated numbly, "I am so sorry, I just can't do it anymore."

Within the week I had two prospective buyers. I chose the one with the most restaurant experience, and negotiated to turn over only the restaurant portion of the lease. I would continue running the marina and collecting the income for the next several years.

The landlord of the property was not pleased with this arrangement, having his eye on the marina income himself. Despite my having to resort to lawyers armed with 'before and after' photos of the place to overcome the landlord's objections, the restaurant was eventually turned over to the new operator relatively smoothly; with the marina remaining my responsibility, and my income.

This was the end of an era for me, and the beginning of a life for Genevieve… for both of us.

'WINDSONG' AND SECRET ISLANDS

Gen and I had outgrown the small villa within a year of moving in. By the third year the walls of the rooms were pushing in on us unbearably, and the lime green kitchen Formica made me want to puke everytime I passed by. When I finally realized we could not live there any more, that we had to have more space and a home of our own, Windsong, the lovely three bedroom house next door to us, with its huge walled garden and hardwood floors, suddenly became vacant.

The minute the tenants told us they were leaving, I negotiated a price with the owner for the property; close to half a million dollars… a price way out of my reach… a price I would have to find a way around.

Very reluctantly I sold my beautiful stone house in France, the one father gave me when he kept his promise to each of his ten children. I hated to sell it, but didn't see any other choice; we needed a house in Nassau, and the banks required a 30% deposit to even contemplate a loan…based on past experience, it never occurred to me to seek help in my ex husband's direction.

"Windsong", the house I coveted, was literally next door to our villa, and owned by the same wealthy Dutchman. He owned another large house on the waterfront nearby, but spent most of his time in Europe. "Windsong" was not on the real-estate market, he only agreed to sell to me because I nagged him to death, and we had become friends over the past few years as neighbors.

The Windsong property included an adjacent two-bedroom cottage; house and cottage separated by twenty feet of garden. I could not afford to buy both places, yet the price I had been given was for the entire property. Via faxes to and from Europe, the Dutchman confirmed he would not sell the house and cottage separately.

Spending $100 for plants to spruce up the cottage's little garden, I placed some pretty pieces of my own furniture in the living room, and brazenly placed a 'for sale' ad for the cottage in the local newspaper. My main goal was to end up with the 3 bedroom house, therefore the price I asked for the cottage was very reasonable considering the desirable Cable Beach area.

In the space of a weekend three couples were ready to put money down on a cottage I did not own. My choice was a couple who were crazy about the place, young and pleasant, and of Bahamian nationality, which would speed up the paperwork and bank loans. Selling to foreigners entailed getting government approval, not necessarily complicated, but often time consuming.

I explained the situation to them thus; "I don't own the property, we will divide it and buy each piece on separate conveyances as part of the same sale, thereby satisfying the owner's requirement of getting paid for the entire property, and having the advantage of saving us money on closing costs".

They gave me a deposit check for $10,000 on the spot, I hired surveyors to split the property the next day, and the sale went ahead with the house going to me and the cottage going simultaneously to them. A good deal for everyone, or as my father would say, *a sixty-sixty deal.*

So Gen and I moved once again, but this time to a happy house. One with richly patinaed wooden floors, bright sunny rooms overlooking that lush, tropical garden, and all within fifty yards of a magnificent beach with access to the flamboyant waterworks and restaurants of the Crystal Palace Hotel. A little private beach in the other direction gave us the choice between being just us, or being part of happy crowds paying top dollar to play for a few days in our backyard.

A home for us to spread out in, to spin in, to dance in. A home for the twelve by eight foot Turkish Nigde Kars carpet living in the trunk of my car for the past two years…the colors and rich texture irresistible to me, avidly participating in a "seized by customs" auction.

Wealthy now, (relatively!) from grueling months spent restoring that decrepit, bankrupt restaurant to the successful waterfront "happening' place it was now, I allowed myself a few tame indulgences. No furs, jewels, or extravagant clothes; just plants, and my exquisite carpet.

That the carpet had been bigger than our villa living room when I bid on it, did not deter me. I knew we would have a house one day worthy of those closely woven threads, a perfect place to show off the *"sweeping indigo central field of this imposing arrangement of powerful geometric motifs from the Nigde knotting region of eastern Anatolia. The beautiful pastel colors derived from leaving the finished carpet in the fierce mountain sun over a considerable period, the soft glow of the pastels contrasting dramatically with the thematic shade of indigo"*… and I quote from the Certificate of Authenticity given me with the purchase of my prize.

It never occurred to me that we would not find a house worthy of this treasure, a house that would tip from spacious to spectacular with this magic carpet poured out over its polished hardwood floors.

Genevieve and I lived happily for three years in this Windsong house, our house. *Relatively* happy I should say, given our twoness instead of threeness. Stronger by now, thinking the worst must be over in our struggle to cope with life on our own, we enjoyed the spaciousness of the house and the lushness of the gardens, the freedom of being together with no pervasive tensions from the restaurant.

I soon started another business. Stored outside in the garden were beautiful Italian tiles waiting patiently over two years for me to tackle the bathroom renovations. Checking to see if they were still usable, I was severely stung by wasps after sticking my hand right into their nest between the tiles. I ran hopping and cursing, hand swelling and throbbing, into the kitchen where I rooted around frantically for the ingredients of the family sting remedy handed down to me by my mother.

The tile man had been helping me sort the tiles. Watching me come out of the house just a few minutes later calmer and quieter, the pain abating, and my hand dripping in a gluey paste, he said in amazement, "You ought to sell that stuff, I've never seen anything work so fast".

I immediately set about creating **"All Better Now"**™. As stated on the label, "A proprietary blend of herbs and powders that draws out insect poison before swelling begins, stopping pain and itching within three to five minutes when applied immediately after being bitten or stung".

The formula was packaged in a compress format, using non-bleached tea bags. The compress only needed to be dampened to activate the healing process.

Three compresses fit perfectly into one small ziplock baggy, easy to grab and ready to use. The individual tea bags could be dipped in either fresh water or salt water, so they were perfect for travel, beach, boat and home First Aid kits.

I designed labels crawling with all manner of cute bugs, bees and jellyfish, on corn yellow paper to catch the eye. The finished product was attractive and effective, and soon we boasted a customer base of hotels and gift shops all over Nassau, and were even asked to set up poolside displays at the brand new Atlantis Resort.

Everyone it seemed, was hungry for a Bahamian product, or any product for that matter that provided relief to customers irritated and upset by contact with jellyfish, mosquitoes and other critter encounters.

The product sold well. We still had the income from the Marina, and life was suddenly so easy compared to the Restaurant days. Now I had time to spend with my Gen girl. All those things mothers take for granted, going to the beach, having lunch together when school was out, going to movies, just relaxing happily as she talked to friends for hours on the phone, life was good. If the other family down the road would let her join in, life would be perfect.

It was still a huge thorn in my side that Gen's dad had given this new wife a lovely life, had adopted her two kids and moved them from public schools to private schools, had given her a beautiful home… Gen's and my home, yet she was still unwilling to accept Genevieve into their family.

It was inconceivable to me that he was not able to ask her to be friendly to his first child. It seemed the most normal thing to me that they should all grow up together. But he never took this stand, saying once, "I would love to spend more time with Genevieve, but not if it means causing trouble at home". What a guy.

* * * * *

Genevieve has a bottomless pit of forgiveness. Always ready to be part of her Dad's family whenever they would have her, she was thrilled to tell me she had baked cookies with the stepmom, that she had been asked to help with dinner, that in a period of relative calm, her stepmother had bought her a skirt.

Gen loved her Daddy, and wanted to see him no matter what. That was one of the prime reasons returning to live in Europe was never an option during these difficult times.

Due to her undaunting perseverance and refusal to give up on her father, a détente had been forged…a few months of bliss broken suddenly by a fight with the older boy that turned into a violent family free for all at her Father's house Christmas Eve, when Gen was twelve.

At seven p.m. on Christmas Eve, she called me on the phone, crying and hysterical; "Pick me up right now! Please Mommy come and get me!"

Hearing the shouting and terrible ruckus in the background, I asked no questions, just raced for the car and got there in four minutes flat. She was sitting in the driveway by the street, outside the closed gate to the property, a sobbing heap under the pile of presents she had so happily carried to their house. The gifts she had taken to put under the tree for each and every one… she and her presents had been thrown out of her Father's house on Christmas Eve.

Unable to bear being in Nassau one minute longer, I called my brother in Malibu. Thank God he was there, his wife and three lovely daughters thrilled to have us stay with them for the Holidays.

The morning flight Christmas day to Los Angeles was empty… people with normal lives were home with their families. Gen and I arrived in Malibu just in time for a perfect Christmas family dinner, and lots of love. Just what the doctor ordered.

We stayed in California throughout the New Year, returning to Nassau armed with the resolution that we would move away, somewhere, anywhere, and find a new life at the first opportunity.

On the trip back we had an extra passenger tucked into a small black duffel bag under the seat, our little puppy, 'Malibu'. The size of a baby Jack Russell, he managed to squirm out of the bag in the middle of the night while everyone was sleeping in the darkened plane, and take a trot back ten rows or so to snuffle around the feet of a woman passenger. Luckily she was too frightened to scream at this warm, furry, unidentified intruder. Instead she wrapped her legs around her neck, stayed in her seat, and buzzed frantically for the stewardess.

I was awakened by a body hunched over in the aisle next to me whispering towards the back of the plane; "You found a WHAT?!" I heard an answering whisper, "It's a puppy!"

I dashed out of my seat and ran back to where a stewardess was holding aloft something small and wriggly. In the seat next to her was the speechless woman in her strange yoga position. I admitted the puppy was mine, thanked the passenger profusely for not screaming, and thereby risking sending the entire plane into panic and chaos. Then Malibu disappeared for the rest of the flight.

The stewardesses were in love with him, kidnapped him, fed him first class tidbits and generally spoiled him rotten. I could barely get him back at the end of the trip.

Genevieve had spied the little bundle of unhappy fur at the Malibu Pet Center the day after Christmas. She begged for this puppy every day for five days, visiting him daily in his cage, the scruffiest inmate in this classy jail. A "pocket dog" she wanted, and at six inches long, he certainly qualified.

I resisted firmly until the sixth day, when Gen made me an offer I couldn't refuse…She promised she would get up for school promptly, and *go to school every day without a hassle* when we got back to Nassau.

The prospect of no more grim morning struggles was like manna from heaven in my frazzled state, and yes, I resorted gladly to bribery and corruption.

It was the best deal I ever made. In the past I was faced every weekday with an unwilling body which I could awaken but not physically wrest from her bed, due to my being several inches and several pounds smaller. My options therefore were limited; tedious persuasion, various forms of motivation, threats…no TV, big deal. Sometimes I was successful and sometimes not.

Now I only had to open her door and toss in the puppy. With a bounce and a wriggle he was on the bed, covering her with puppy kisses and love. She would wake with a smile on her face, and true to her word get up and ready for school without any struggle at all for the last two terms. To me it was a miracle.

In our minds we knew we were out of Nassau once school was over. We would look seriously for a new place to live over the summer. But where would we go? We loved California, but it was a huge move with all the animals, and I never had my father's energy. It would be expensive too. Fort Lauderdale is another favorite place but still a big upheaval.

I didn't know where to look, didn't know where to begin, but always had my brain in search mode, on the lookout for a sign. In

July I found our secret island. I was called there for a Restaurant consulting job. I can only guess Someone in the great scheme of things was looking out for us.

By August I had found a tenant for Windsong, and on a weekend visit to Hopetown to find a place to rent, I walked straight into the only cottage available for yearly rental. Weekly rentals were becoming a growing source of income for many of the local residents, and more lucrative than an annual rental, however the offer of six months rent in advance was an offer the owner did not refuse.

Perched on a little hill above a tiny beach, Lavender Cottage as I was to call it, faced the pretty harbor entrance, western sunsets, and a small private Island at the mouth of the harbor, Eagle Rock. Strangely the little house guarding Eagle Rock two years later became the property of the friend crucial to my introduction to Hopetown. Who could have guessed that the next few years would see us trekking back and forth at low tide between her island and my cottage…for a cup of tea and a chat.

When Gen and I moved in September from Nassau to Hopetown, it was a much smaller group than my parent's momentous odyssey from Malibu to France. Only one child, three dogs, two birds, and a cat, but a feat of organization nonetheless; moving from a large three bedroom house to a two bedroom cottage previously used for weekly rentals…with *not one* closet.

To accommodate this little zoo, we traveled via chartered plane. The dogs hopped up the steps like old pros, and behaved quite calmly in the spaces created for them by taking out a row of seats. The Captain was also quite relaxed when midflight, our large black Retriever sort of hound, Pepper, stuck his cold nose on the back of his neck and gave him a reassuring lick to tell him he was doing a great job. None of the dogs were in cages, just on good behavior.

Well two thirds of them were behaving. Our little Malibu dog was very concerned with finding a way into the cockatiel's cage, strapped into a seat next to him. They were both at the same level now, and Mal was determined to have a few feathers despite my warnings of dire consequences. In his hunting, stalking mode, with nose pressed hard against the apprehensive bird's cage, he was quite oblivious to the vibration and noise of our takeoff, and in fact the entire flight, he never left his post for a moment. He is very tenacious. I covered the cage with a towel, so at least the bird didn't have to see those intense little eyes the entire trip.

The ferry from Marsh Harbour on the mainland of Abaco to our little Island was chartered also, so the dogs were allowed onboard as on the plane… leashes only, no cages. They had rarely ever been in the car, let alone in a cage. It would have been as traumatic for me as for them, thus the charters were worth the extra expense.

Like several of the more recent cottages on this island, ours was built with short term, weekly or monthly visits in mind, not annual rentals. But still…NO closets?! How's a girl to manage? Luckily one of Gen's friends from a previous visit to the island turned out to be very handy with carpenter's tools. In a flash we each had a roomy closet. Our relatively small bedrooms were now reduced to 'barely there', but we were happy. Seventy or so boxes of 'indispensable items', and still a houseful of furniture back in Nassau…where did all this STUFF come from?

We didn't care about the lack of space, we were so thrilled to be on our own, away from the maddening crowd, and with a spectacular vista at every window.

The private school on the mainland proved to be a first; the first time since she was three that Gen was *happy to go to school,* the first time she felt like joining in on special yearbook and debate projects, the first time we felt happy chatting in the morning getting a lunch box ready, the first time she felt so good about things I get a daily happy hug and a kiss before she heads on foot to the ferry dock for the fifteen minute boat ride to school.

As the student-laden ferry passes by our porch on its way out of the harbor, there is a hand waving that is discernable amidst the friendly chaos of forty school kids. This is the first time without *dread* of any kind for both of us.

* * * * *

Our Malibu puppy was also blissfully happy in our new Island cottage. Barely reaching the elbows of the other two dogs, he rides roughshod over the much bigger hounds. Pepper and Cinnamon, silly names given to puppies by Gen when she was seven and we rescued them from the Nassau pound. Large, floppy retriever types, brothers in fact, one black and solid like a bear, the other gold and white, with a circus dog personality. Cinnamon is happy to climb onto a surfboard with or without Gen; a comical surfer who even with four feet, can't maintain his balance very long. With a toothy grin and tail wagging happily, he tolerates hats, sunglasses or any other foolishness Gen decides to try out on him.

The big dogs love the water, heading out into the mouth of the harbor in front of our porch like two seals. At high tide Malibu waits not so patiently at the shoreline, well aware his short little legs are no match for theirs in this medium. At low tide the three of them frolic on the exposed sandbar, not ten feet from the deep channel into the harbor. This sight astonishes incoming boats, suddenly realizing how narrow the channel must be.

At very low spring tides the dogs romp right out to Eagle Rock, the small private island just beyond the sandbar and to the right of the harbor entrance, where they play Robinson Caruso… in the days before the island acquired a resident.

They check out the uninhabited house perched atop the rocky hill, with its three empty windows staring at me as I write, then race twice around the little island to rustle up the seagulls and send them squawking into the air. Finally the obligatory quick pee on the small upside down boat drawn up on the shore, before splashing happily back to our cottage.

I have included a small sketch of the sandbar, the cottage and the harbor mouth where incoming dolphins sometimes meet outgoing dogs, as it is difficult to portray in words this small area of activity.

Leaving the harbor, the channel curves in front of our cottage and heads out to the Sea of Abaco, a relatively protected body of water between our island and the mainland, fifteen minutes away by boat. Behind the cottage, walking in the opposite direction away from the harbor, we pass the ballpark where even on the hottest days kid and adult teams vie for glory.

Up a sandy dune we pass through the beautiful old cemetery dating back to the early 1800's; the stone tombs lie above the ground in various states of disarray. Here a headstone has cracked and toppled over, there a Casuarina tree grows straight and true to the sky, right through the center of someone's ancestors, the tomb having no choice but to split in two. Dust to dust.

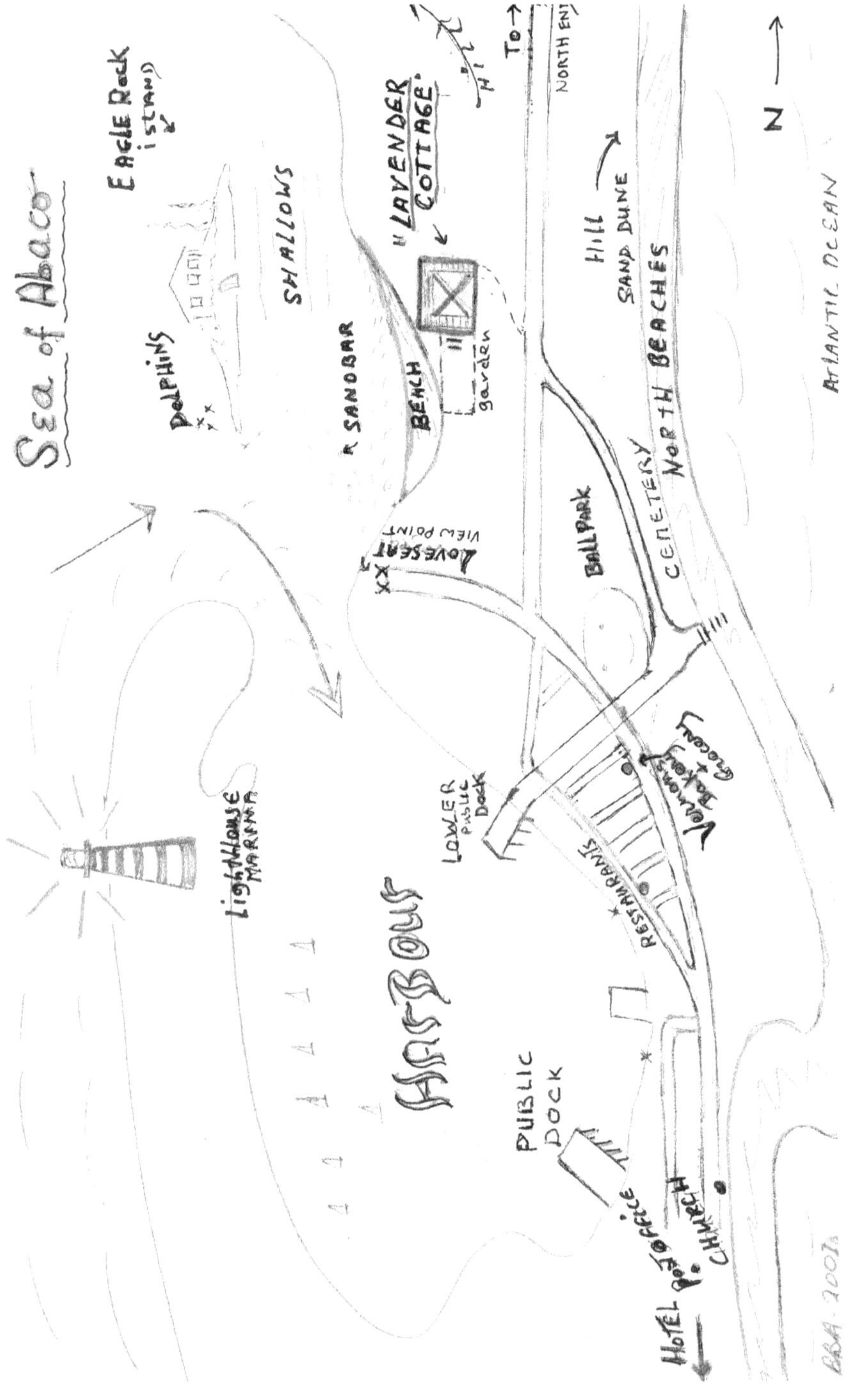
Sea of Abaco
Eagle Rock
i stand
Dolphins
Shallows
Sandbar
Beach
"Lavender Cottage"
garden
Hill
To →
North End
Hill
Sand Dune
North Beaches
N
Atlantic Ocean
Loveseat
View Point
Ballpark
Cemetery
Lower Public Dock
Lighthouse Marina
Harbour
Restaurants
Public Dock
Hotel
Post Office
Church
BBA 2002

Reaching the top of the hill, your breath suddenly leaves you. Where there was only sand and grass but a second ago, the Atlantic Ocean has burst out of nowhere, right in your face. It sweeps past reefs teeming with tropical treasures, out to the horizon in colors of indigo blue, turquoise, aqua, lavender. Gifts for the senses of sight, sound, and smell. For the sense of touch, there is another present at the bottom of the dune, a very spectacular beach.

A postcard beach. Two miles or so of it, where white crests ride waves of lime sherbet from the reef to the shore, crashing at your feet in powerful sprays of froth.

All three dogs go crazy on this endless beach, chasing real and imaginary birds back and forth at top speed, little Malibu somehow making up for his short legs by amazing bursts of speed, ears pinned back against his head by the G forces. The two big dogs stop only to swim and catch a wave or two, bodysurfing in their own doggy way, with the joy of excited children. Two friendly happy dogs, with a bad secret.

They get a real thrill out of chasing people. The excitement of Nassau, the screams of terror as bodies of would-be robbers scrabbled over our walls to get away from their gnashing teeth is still with these dogs. They are Nassau dogs and their protectiveness was welcome there.

How many times in the last few years did I awake in the night to the sounds of running feet crashing through the lush foliage of our Nassau garden? To the curses of fast moving bodies hurtling towards the high native stone wall that surrounded the property. Bodies that without the dogs, would still be pulling out the louvers of our windows, or sawing through the protective bars before boldly climbing into the house to rob us, the noise of their nocturnal activity softened by the hum of the airconditioners. How many times? So often that I didn't even bother to call the police.

Here on our new friendly little island this aggressive mode is no longer necessary. We are therefore having a crash course in being nice, being laid back, and NOT barking at strangers.

Old thrills die hard however, and for peace of mind I have built a high picket fence around the garden next to our cottage, and rejoice in the knowledge that the island population is safe.

While the fence was being completed the dogs all spent a week *inside* the cottage. A stretch for me, as the place is small enough without two large furry bodies and one small one. Two sets of wagging tails sweeping everything off the coffee table several times a day. The third tail couldn't reach.

In spite of the inconvenience, we got along because the payoff was something I would have otherwise missed. Very early every morning they awakened me with gentle snuffles outside my bedroom door, getting me up in time to catch the first dawn's light on the water… different from any other time of day, and not really something I have words to describe. Silver maybe. Silver and glinting, glinting on dark colorless water, as in a black and white print…all outline and silhouette and no color.

Never would it have occurred to me to raise my body out of bed at that hour by choice, but I could not be annoyed by their pre dawn eagerness to be out in the cool air, it was just too beautiful.

Thus it came to pass early one morning that I was writing a letter by hand outside on the porch, my computer lifeless and sad. The local power company had decided once again, for reasons unknown to us its lowly customers, that it would be fun to turn off the electricity for an indeterminate amount of time.

To me this was no hardship, particularly when I conjure up images of what it must have been like for Shakespeare and his fellow geniuses, creating their meticulous masterpieces with only quill and ink. The difficulty I have is of a different variety, keeping my mind on the paper.

Suddenly a flash of white skims across the water, begging my full attention. The horizontal blur changes shape midair, stops, and slides into the water to become a vertical white statue, motionless, too beautiful to be real. A sculptured Great Heron planted in the ripples lapping the edge of my little beach. The rest of the world fades away, we eye each other a full minute, his metal feathers glinting in the sun.

I too remain motionless, frozen yet watchful. The golden beak tapered to a finite angle never quivers. Then the sharp black eyes relax, now seem strangely trusting. I have been reviewed, I have been inspected, I have been absorbed… I have been found not too frightening.

The Heron shrugs himself back to a living thing, lifts a long, long leg to start an unhurried stroll, then quick as a flash that sharp beak is holding breakfast, a hapless little fish that was no match for the fierce thrust of the long flexible neck, down which it now slides. The Heron gives me another piercing look, and a nod that means "adieu."

Without a flutter or flap, there is silent liftoff. Effortless, controlled, those powerful wings carry my living sculpture away. For a very long moment the shoreline seems empty and lifeless. Then the movement of the water beckons to me, a reminder that this is a good time to complete my letter, before another startling vision takes me off to a different magic place.

A constant distraction is our sandbank. When it is submerged at high tide, the bar of sand in the shallower water is still visible to me from my porch or windows, but it must be invisible to boats in the entrance channel at certain times of the day. It is a rare week that at least two or three rental speedboats don't land on it with a shock, and a roaring complaint from the misused outboard engines…amateur captains trying to cut between my house and the little island in front of me instead of going around to the channel, with predictable results.

The embarrassed maneuverings of the macho driver, trying to look cool while his boat is obviously going nowhere, is always a source of amusement to me. It's a wonder I get anything done at all.

Some of the captains cleverly back off, while others resort to the less glamorous but effective tactic of jumping onto the sandbar or knee-high water, and pull or push the boat until it abruptly hits the deep channel water. The shouts of laughter from others in the boat as the pullee/pushee suddenly disappears underwater are priceless. It is also fun watching their efforts to clamber back onboard from the deep water. It takes very little to amuse me these days.

The mystery to me is the sailboats. When a sailboat goes aground coming or going through the narrow channel, and they often do; no matter how many men are on board, no matter that a man is at the helm and three are at the bow, if there is a woman on board, it is somehow her fault. I can hear the yelling from here… "Helen you idiot, why didn't you tell me." "Susan, what the hell is that! Now what are we going to do?" "Linda, you blankety blank, are you blind?!" etc. etc.

The women silently and stoically wait for the storm of abuse to pass (I have never heard **one** yell back). Sometimes it is so bad I want to wade out there with a big sign that says, "Where were YOU when you went aground - you obnoxious loudmouth?!"

I don't know where these men go after they get safely in the harbor, sometimes hours later depending on the whim of the tide that left them aground, or who they turn into when walking around town, as everyone is as pleasant as can be, and you never hear a rude word anywhere.

MOI, IN THE BEVERLY HILLS JAIL

Well, I have written and written, and still my Gen girl is not home. Once again I thank God for this safe island Paradise we live in. It is nine o'clock. Her curfew is ten, if she is not back by then I will go and look for her. At least I have a Plan. Making a plan quiets the stomach.

It is Plans that have kept us going through these years of turbulence; plans to move, plans to build, plans to make money, plans to travel, plans to be more consistent in dealings with my daughter. Without a plan I am like a ship without a rudder, foundering in uncharted waters.

I find I have left the family in France to its own devices for many pages. This is a good time to return to the giant stones, the ferns unfurling in the mist, the crisp air, the wine harvests; and if the mood strikes, a bit about my months in South Africa, and a short stint in a Beverly Hills jail.

Perhaps by then my sweet girl will be home.

If Father wasn't writing, he was inventing, Delving into toy designing with his trademark enthusiasm and delight, he came up with a winner marketed by Ohio Art; the Busy Buzz Buzz was a pen in the shape of a vibrating bee that produced swirling lines… the forerunner of the ever popular "Spirograph Pens".

Several of his imaginative designs were for Benson children only; a magnificent Sunflower Shower, six feet tall and flowering in the bottom of the castle garden, its solid plastic frame camouflaged by authentic garden colors of sunshine yellow and earlyleaf green.

The Sunflower faced skyward, forming a shallow basin that filled up maddeningly slowly with cool water on a hot summer day. Kids circled below, expectant faces upturned with glee and dread... then the overfill, tipping the precarious balance of the Sunflower, showering all below amid shrieks and giggles.

There are similar summer garden water toys on the market now, but this was years ago, when our Sunflower Shower was the only one of its kind...and how the little ones loved it.

Father had the giant fireplaces at Chaban burning nonstop in fall, winter and early spring, no doubt counting on their great attraction and warmth to evaporate memories of the California sun shining far, far away. While the fires were intensely beautiful and hot, I distinctly remember why I abandoned ship that first September and headed for Rome.

Standing before the great dry logs crackling and throwing off tremendous heat, a great deal of comfort was to be had only on one side of the body, that side offered to the flames. If it was the backside, the front side received no benefit, and vice versa.

A constant rotation of the body was therefor deployed, rather like a chicken on a rotisserie spit, and as long as one was within ten feet of the fireplace, everything was toasty.

It is hard to live like that though, glued to the fireplace. There are perfectly viable reasons one has to move away from the fire from time to time...to cook, to eat, to help get the kids ready for school, to pee, to go to bed; and that was the killer.

Getting up the nerve to race away from the fire, cross acres of cold parquet floor as quickly as possible, dash up miles of stairs, shedding clothes at the speed of light, to jump into freezing flannel pajamas, then into equally icy sheets, was a nightly trauma before I moved to Italy and the nunnery; where hot water in the faucets and the fireplaces I took for granted at Chaban haunted my sleepless nights.

Father was in his element designing ways to get the heat from the fires into the rooms…yards of pipe wound round the backs of the chimneys to carry the hot air to unknown directions; fans were installed to blow the heat towards us instead of up the chimney… along with the soot and ash.

Pipes ran along the spaces beneath the floors, theoretically carrying warm air to all the rooms. Long flat cushions, like fat brown snakes, were placed at the base of doors to keep the heat inside. All to no avail, we still froze our backsides off.

Finally one winter visit father had it under control. He simply borrowed a solution from a Sears catalog, and ordered dozens of electric blankets. Now a quick dash to our rooms half an hour before bedtime to turn on that wonderful little switch, pajamas warming up nicely under the covers… a small fire glowing in the hearth… and going to bed in winter suddenly became the best part of the day.

With the daylight hours getting shorter and the summer air turning to brisk September, it was time to head back to Paris and my job, with weekends at Chaban whenever I felt I could handle the drive.

Sometimes my boss Mark would join me. He was roughly father's age, and they formed a mutual appreciation society as soon as I introduced them. It was in his office that Maritee and I met, became friendly, and decided to become roommates… in the days before she became Father's roommate.

Mark never missed a Vendange weekend. In late September or early October, friends gathered from all corners of the globe; from nearby castles in France, from Switzerland and England, from Malibu; they would all drop what they were doing to come to the Dordogne to help pick grapes... and party.

Out in the fields from early morning when it was still cool, we picked basketloads of sweet red grapes and dumped them into barrels waiting by the side of the country road. Then we stomped on them, the kids literally climbing into the barrels and dancing on the grapes, compressing them in the smaller portable vats, before transport to the castle farm via tractordrawn wagon. I have lost a wonderful old photo of Roland, my hunky boyfriend you met in Greece, stomping around in the barrels with my little brothers, boots up to his knees slick with grapejuice, a great big handsome kid playing with the little kids in the squished grapes.

At the farm the mashed grapes were poured into huge vats ten feet high and fifteen wide to begin the transformation from mash and stems...resplendent with bugs, spiders and all manner of living protein straight from the vine, to the magnificent crystal clear wine we produced the first few years we were in residence.

The picking and stomping was the "work" part of the weekend, the rest was the eating, drinking and dancing that took place in the ballroom. Tables laid out for fifty or so guests, roaring fire in the huge hearth, and local musicians hired for most of the night. Medieval revelry at its best.

* * * * *

Two, three years of Paris and its weather was enough for me. I've been too long in the shadow of those majestic but gray, gray stone buildings. Despite the weekend breaks to the countryside, my heart begins to long for sunshine and the tang of salt on the lips. I have a craving for the California life again.

And Roland is driving me crazy. Handsome, sweet, funny, (I think I have said all those things, and all those things he is), but driving me crazy nonetheless. And I am driving him crazy, prodding him relentlessly to make something of himself, when all he wants is a nice bottle of wine, a good piece of Brie and me… or a good piece of me and some Brie.

The day he tried to strangle me, then threw me in a bathtub, but still would not leave me, would not move out of my apartment; that was the day I decided it was time to high tail it out of Paris while I still had all my body parts intact.

Unwilling to part with my Alfa, I found I could ship it from Paris to Los Angeles for $1,000, which I thought was very reasonable. Done, and I am off.

The car and I arrived within a week of one another; me bright eyed and ready for more adventures, my pretty Alfa dusty and forlorn on the dock, but intact. She was soon shining and humming again, and we embarked on the search for an apartment and a job. A girlfriend from Paris was now living in California, and invited me to stay with her while I organized my life. Two weeks after I arrived in Los Angeles, Roland showed up at our front door. How he found me, I do not know.

Contrite, determined to have me back, willing to work as a restaurant dishwasher if he had to (the only job he could find as an illegal Frog) and handsome as hell, my girlfriend swooned and said he could stay with us for two weeks. He did try, he did get a job, he did study English diligently, he was as pleasant and kind as could be, but I was over him, so very over him.

I do love him for coming back from his horrible dishwashing job one day and asking me, "What is a pedxing?". Taxing my brain to the max, I could think of no such word in the English language. "Where did you see it?" I asked.

"On the road, over some big white stripes".

It hit me then, ped. xing., *Pedestrian Crossing*. It sort of broke my heart, it was so cute. But there was no future for us…I sent him back to Paris with love.

Finding an apartment was easy, I loved it immediately. It was just like being in France; a big sunny living room, an alcove bedroom, wood floors and high ceilings, tucked away just off Rodeo Drive in Beverly Hills. Six apartments around a courtyard with trees and shade, French windows and a price I could afford, if only I had a job.

I asked the landlord to hold the apartment for me for a week, and somehow talked a large construction company into giving me an office job. I say somehow, because I did not have U.S citizenship or a green card, and I don't remember being qualified for anything except talking in several languages and getting done whatever was asked of me.

I must have done something right as I was there for two years, the company having kindly sponsored the application for my first green card. I have had two or three over the years, losing them with extended stays in Europe and forgetting to fill out the required paperwork to keep them up to date.

You may wonder if I gave Roberto a call now that we were in the same country. Well, no. Shortly after he left Paris, I met Roland, and when he moved in with me, I sent Roberto's lovely antique sapphire and diamond engagement ring back to him via a friend passing through Paris. The ring was beautiful, but it never occurred to me to keep his family heirloom... I was the one bailing out.

So I did not call Roberto, but heard of him through friends. The woman he married built up a successful business originating from the romantic notes they left around the house for one another; "Love Is...", perhaps you remember seeing those little notes in all the stores for a few years, or you may have even sent one to someone.

I don't remember any particular man at this point in my life in California, perhaps I was on a sabbatical, just enjoying catching up with chums from my Malibu and Marymount days, and meeting lots of new faces. After two years with the construction company, one of my girlfriends announced she was getting married to a football star, Paul Hornung, and would I like to take over her job at Twentieth Century Fox Studios working for a Producer? I was sorry to leave my kind employers, but who could resist? The interview was in the producer's office on the Studio lot, and all went well. I was asked to start the following Monday.

Getting up extra early on Monday morning, I dressed in my chicest Gucci, Pucci and Mucci, jumped in my shiny red Alfa, and with plenty of time to spare headed out on the short drive from my pretty apartment to the Studio... and somehow caught the eye of an early bird cop.

I don't remember what my slight infraction was, or if in fact there was one other than being a blonde in a bright red car, but as a general policy, California licenses in the hands of a cop are subject to a ritual computer check. Returning from his car with my license and a grim look on his face, he said without preamble, "park your car, you are under arrest."

"What on earth for?" I asked, more astounded than upset.

"There is a warrant for your arrest for an unpaid traffic violation several years ago." This was altogether possible; when the family moved to Europe, paying a ticket would have been the last thing on my mind.

I refused to leave the Alfa on the side of the road, and took pains to park in the safest spot I could find, which required the arresting officer to hold up traffic for my maneuverings…I got a small measure of happiness out of making him do my bidding . Asked politely to get into the police car, it still seemed such a lark that I did not even object when my hands were handcuffed behind my back… although I did think it was a bit of overkill. When we walked into the police station however, and other people started to look at me, hands cuffed behind my back, with that "what did SHE do?" look, I realized this was no joke.

A heat wave washed over me as the cuffs became claustrophobic. Not letting on that I was about to go into panic mode, I calmly talked the cop into undoing them, restoring minimally my dignity, and was allowed to make not one, but two phone calls.

The first was to an old boyfriend to bail me out (all this for a $68 ticket!) and the second to my new boss, with surely the least heard excuse in the annals of stupid "why I'm late" excuses…

"Hi" I said, "I'll be a bit late… I'm in jail."

Like every boss I have ever had until I became my own boss, he was understanding, kind, and amused by me, and our relationship did not suffer one bit for my being a jailbird.

And a wonderful job it was. Reading scripts, writing synopses of them, arranging meetings between writers, directors and actors. Mel Brooks had an office just down the hall, James Caan would stop by often to see my boss, and I was regularly invited to parties at Hefner's mansion, where I met Hugh O'Brien…of Wyatt Earp fame for those of you old enough to remember. Although Hugh had quite a few years on me, he turned out to be a good friend and a fun date for several months.

Interesting people flowed through 'Wyatt's' house in Benedict Canyon like leaves on a lazy stream, swirling and eddying together for a moment in time, then floating off in their own direction. Maureen Dean and I played pool together several times, and it was through a mutual friend of ours that I snagged my Studio job. This was before Watergate, and seeing Mo later standing by her man John in court on TV was a source of amazement to us all.

This was my Hollywood era. Shortly before meeting Wyatt Earp, I spent a day in the desert with Steve McQueen. 'Platonically' I now rather regret to say, playing with dune buggys and big motorcycles.

We met in a nightclub on Rodeo Drive. I was with a group of friends when a bearded guy suddenly appeared at our table and asked me to dance. I was about to decline politely when my date surprised me by saying jovially, "Sure Steve", and told me to go ahead. After a couple of dances 'Steve' brought me back to the table, said "thanks" to me and my date, and left. Puzzled, I asked, "What was that all about, why did you want me to dance with him?"

He replied "Don't you know who that was?"

"No, I thought it must be a friend of yours."

When he told me who it was, we had a good chuckle. Steve did not ask for my number that night, but called the next day (Hollywood magic?)... a nice change from those whose trademark it is to swear they will call, then disappear into the gloaming. He asked me out. We spent the day in the desert. A really great day. His friends arrived in fancy busses and trucks with their fancy bikes, and music blared from huge speakers set up on top of the busses. Steve was both attentive and macho.

That would have satisfied most girls, but I also liked conversation. Steve was all bikes and beer, that day anyway, and had a little trouble hearing my soft voice, I can't remember whether due to the loud music or previous gun noise injuries. I was shocked when he passed away a few years later, but glad to have the memory.

One day a strikingly beautiful woman came into the office and we had a chat while she waited for my boss. Anne was an aspiring actress, who later became the wife of Richard Harris. Strangely enough Richard was to come into my life years later in Nassau, when he leased a dock at the restaurant Marina. His house across the Harbor on Paradise Island had no road access.

There was no way I could know, as she was sitting in my office in Beverly Hills talking about her boyfriend Richard, that her Richard would one day years later eat at my Restaurant in Nassau, and quite often too, accompanied by his two little white dogs, which he carried around tucked into the top of his standard attire, white cotton overalls. With his white hair, white outfit, and the white dogs with their four black button eyes peering out of his chest, he was a funny sight until you got close enough to see what was going on.

This was in one of Richard's non-drinking periods. He and Anne had by now been married, divorced, and become friends again. He was always a wonderful guest, full of interesting stories, and happy to sign autographs when customers asked me if it was all right to approach him. This was a time of new recognition for Richard, having just completed and excellent film whose title I cannot for the life of me remember.

Only on one occasion did the Hostess call me at home on one of my rare nights off to say, "Mr. Harris is dancing on a table and is quite drunk". I asked if the other customers minded, and she said, "No, they are enjoying it".

"Well then" I said, "Just keep an eye on him and make sure he doesn't hurt himself, and get him down as soon as you can". My wonderful hostess Donnell, she was the best.

It seems I am somehow back at the restaurant, although I thought we were well finished with that, but given Regis Philbin's great success, I am happy to include this little anecdote.

Regis and his family showed up for lunch at Captain Nemo's unannounced one day, and had such a good time he mentioned it on his morning TV show on their return to New York. He would be pleased to know we had calls for months thereafter for reservations for "The very same table where Regis Philbin had eaten."

The next week he sent a postcard to thank me for a lovely lunch, adding something about having tripped over a low chain at the entrance to the dock… I knew he was referring to the one I had put there to stop taxis from driving onto the dock. He said he hurt his shoulder, but made a joke of it and promised not to sue, for which I thank him.

And now we are truly out of Nassau, back in Beverly Hills, and heading to France. After three years at my fun job at 20th Century

Fox Studios, my producer moved on to something else and out of his Studio office. I sold my sweet Alfa and headed back to France. Three years anywhere seemed to be my limit, perhaps that is a Gemini thing.

OF MONKS AND MYSTICS

At certain times of the year, on moonlit nights and in the very early mornings, the valleys below Chaban disappear. In their place are clouds so thick and billowy white, that you must stop yourself from stepping out onto them; so strongly convinced are you that walking from one mountain top to the other across this beckoning white softness would take nothing more than the will to do so.

Chaban sits atop a mountain crest. In the first rays of dawn, not a trace can be seen of the two narrow tarmac roads winding up either side of the densely forested mountain, until the roads pop out of the mist to meet and merge at the top, forming a narrow, mile long plateau running the length of the mountain top. The perfect French valleys below are still invisible. This thick blanket of cotton must turn into fog and lift away before we can see the beauty of the silvery river below, winding past sleepy villages; see the patchwork squares of different crops forming a postcard perfect farmland quilt.

By moonlight, with the clouds lapping at the edge of the plateau, the valley becomes a glowing white sea, irresistible to passing ghost canoes paddling silently, gliding effortlessly across this giant lake in the sky. Valley of the Clouds, Valley of Illusion.

As the morning unfolds, the fog lazily climbs the remaining distance to the top of the mountain, surrounding the lower realms of Chaban in a mystical moat. The Castle remains tall and haughty, impervious to the kisses of the wispy tendrils reaching up to shyly toy with the golden stones of the lower walls, warmed now by the first rays of the sun.

Sensing its advances rejected, admitting that swarming the tower is now impossible in the direct light of day, the fog retreats, spilling down over the hilltop pastures, rolling like a wave across wild grass and flowers. The grazing horses lose their legs, casually levitating a while before disappearing completely in the fog.

One thousand now invisible acres stretch away from the castle in all directions; pastures to the south, truffle oaks to the west, vineyards to the east, devoured by the fog as if they never existed. Yet all is not silent, all is not still.

Underneath the undulating gray blanket there is a hustle and bustle in the surrounding forests.

One of the first things Father attended to when he bought the property of Chateau de Chaban, was to arrange with the Mayors of the three neighboring townships to designate the property a "Reserve Biologique"; a heavily posted "No Hunting" area that would become a sanctuary for fauna and flora… the deer, boar, pheasants and their kin now finally safe from the rush of madmen and their baying dogs during hunting season.

The wild animals loved their sanctuary. Although unfenced, they somehow sensed the boundaries of the property. Deer could often be seen grazing with the horses early mornings and at dusk, and we all had to be warned to stay away from the wild pigs with their cute little piglets. The protective sow, with her sharp beady eyes, was at her most dangerous then.

Our 'reserve biologique' was of course not very popular with the local hunters, and it was years before they grudgingly gave up on their favorite hunting grounds. Without fail the first day of hunting season we would find them parked on the side of the hilltop lane, guns in hand. While not trespassing directly onto the property, they blatantly sent their hunting dogs into the protected area to roust out the game and drive it towards them.

Enforcing the law was tricky; arresting dogs was not on the agenda, and the hunters were invariably villagers related to people working for us at the castle.

Over time a sort of peace prevailed. We trapped a few of their dogs, kept them for a few days, (beautiful, smart dogs they were), extracting promises from their embarrassed owners to hunt elsewhere from now on before returning their dogs, baying and tails a wagging.

I wish I could say life was peaceful for all the animal residents, but in a nightmare accident, our pretty bay filly from California did not fare so well as the suicidal bay of earlier chapters. One exceptionally cold foggy morning kept me in my cozy bed as long as possible. Suddenly I was shocked out of a peaceful reverie by piercing screams, coming from outside the Castle.

Jumping to the window I saw nothing, literally nothing. The fog was so thick the fields below were completely invisible, yet the screams were real, screams of terror, desperation. Racing downstairs in my pajamas, no time for clothes, I reached the outside doors at the same time as Father and three or four other members of the household, I have no idea which ones, just in time to see my younger sister Anne materialize out of the fog, sobbing and screaming, incoherent, pointing out to the middle of the pasture.

Telling her to wait with the other kids, Father and I headed into the fog, making it only twenty feet before seeing a trail of blood on the ground, a lot of blood. With the sobbing in the background getting fainter as the smothering fog absorbed all sound, we pushed forward. The trail was easy to follow, too easy, but the fog was so thick we could only see three feet ahead of us. We moved carefully, silently, physically pushing back the damp grayness that seemed to strangle us, made it hard to breathe. Moving faster now, the red trail mesmerizing us, calling to us to hurry…terrified to think what we could possibly find at the end of this journey into a cold gray hell.

Running now, we seemed to be going in crazy circles, up and down hills, the trail turning into a constant stream of blood. How could there be so much blood? The silence was deafening when suddenly we heard her. Came upon her wheezing her last breaths. Prone on her side, a wooden stake through her heart.

Impossible to speak, we patted her in a vain attempt at some kind of comfort. Did she hear us? Did she care? I don't know, it was years ago and I still get sick thinking of it.

My little sister was inconsolable. Only twelve or thirteen at the time, she blamed herself for tying the filly to a stake in the fence instead of the riding rail. Nothing could make her hear our feeble arguments that the law of averages should have made it impossible for a horse to jerk a stake out of a fence, and still tied to it, trot off with it swinging in front of her; attached to it in such a way that if she cantered up a hill at just a certain angle, then fell on the stake at just the wrong moment, the weight of her body would push it through her chest and into her heart.

We know horses are capable of getting into the most improbable situations, yet because they are so big it is easy to forget they need our protection. A hard way to learn the lesson.

* * * * *

With winter soon approaching, Father and Maritee felt a craving to live in Hawaii for six months. They put me in charge of the estate during their absence, affording me the perfect opportunity to delve into the project of sorting out the details of the 'donation' of property to the Tibetan Lamas, and the houses gifted to the Benson offspring.

The children needed the deeds to their houses and land, the monk's property had to be defined and title turned over to them, and the chateau had to be separated from the donation of property so that Father, Maritee and their three little girls would have somewhere to live. Yes, in his enthusiasm to divest of worldly goods, Father had given the castle away also. I separated Chaban from the donation, and do not remember if or how he explained this to the Tibetans.

Once the children's houses and the castle were removed from the property being given away, there was still plenty of land for the Tibetans to go along with their beautiful stone farmhouse. Acres and acres of land… vineyards and forests, beautiful fields and pastures with the proverbial brook running through them, hills and valleys.

One particular valley I have such fond memories of. As kids we would trek down the hill from the castle past the little stone house that would one day be mine, to the stream at the bottom of the valley.

We would picnic there amongst the wildflowers, seated on a great quilt surrounded by crusty loaves of hot bread from the bakery half a mile away, thick slices of ham, pate, and cheeses that make my mouth water just thinking of them now. After a lazy lunch, a little nap, and a frolic in the stream, there were blackberries to pick all the way back up the winding path to the Castle.

I love that pretty little piece of land. I couldn't know at the time I would now yearn for my daughter to have just that little piece of France for picnics with her children when I am long gone.

It was an enormous task sorting through the deeds and parcel numbers of hundreds of acres spread across three different townships; Le Moustier, Plazac, and St. Leon Sur Vezere, each with their own registry office.

As much as I admired the Lamas for their healing powers and knowledge, it was a daily struggle to resign myself to giving away our perfect picnic spot, those acres of vineyards, the valley pastures, and priceless hilltop sites to these guests of father's. Tibetans who would henceforth pave the way for the Buddhist traditions to flourish in this corner of France.

Difficult to give these luscious acres away knowing Father could sell only a small portion and live his last years a wealthy man. Or better yet, he could leave those magnificent acres to us, his children.

The bottom line argument I consoled myself with was this; "He is giving us each a house as he promised, and it is his property to do with as he likes."

That was my reasoning, my consolation, as I signed away pieces of green worth a prince's ransom.

Before leaving for Hawaii, father had gone on a business trip to Paris. On his return he brought in his wake an angel disguised as an architect. In his early twenties, soft spoken and gentle, radiant blue eyes full of warmth and humor… in the social desert of the French countryside, I was immediately smitten.

The attraction was mutual, and when father and Maritee left for Hawaii the architect and I couldn't have been happier. Time sped as we loved and laughed, and amazingly, did a lot of work.

This young architect's unlikely mandate was to furnish preliminary drawings for a Monastery building that would suit the cultural and architectural requirements of the Tibetans, currently living in the beautiful stone farm house a mile from the castle, without shocking the equilibrium of the French countryside.

Visiting the Lamas on a break from creating order in the chaos of my deeds and maps, it came to my attention that with the fall rains, the road to their dwelling was becoming a muddy, impassable trail.

The walkway from the hilltop road to the entrance of the Lama's farmhouse was a distance of approximately three hundred feet. Visitors from all over Europe, the U.S. and even South Africa were tromping through in order to share a brief moment with a real Tibetan Lama. French visitors arrived also, many of them with their children, mistakenly looking for a glimpse of the four-legged variety of llama.

The nearby French villagers were the last to succumb to the unique charm of the monks, many of them by virtue of their pocketbook, as business in these quiet villages had never been so good. The bakeries were doing record sales in croissants, crusty loaves and pain-au-chocolat, and the small hotels were fully booked during months they normally would be closed.

As father was away and funds for paving the path were not in the budget, I devised a plan to build a road, a solid, natural looking lane. A plan that would kill two birds with many stones. The adjacent pasture was full of stones that needed clearing. We could toss the medium size stones from the pasture onto the deep mud of the path to stabilize the worst of the sloppy stuff. With the help of the many hands living near the Lamas, I calculated this would be quick work.

On the castle property was a sand quarry just full of dark yellow sand with traces of clay…the perfect mixture I thought, to pour in tractorloads over the rocks and mud. I was sure the sand would absorb the mud and bind to it. My plan was then to roll something heavy over the mud, rocks, clay and sand by whatever means possible, creating a hard, smooth, durable surface.

I thought the plan was excellent. We had to build the entrance road quickly before the rainstorms began in earnest. The problem was there was no '*We*'… the many hands were not forthcoming. The material was free and there for the taking, only the labor was lacking.

There was much scoffing from the students living on the premises at the Tibetan Center, translating and shopping for them.. that "a road could not be built without tar or asphalt, that it would never last, that the first rain would wash it away", yak yak yak. (pardon the pun; llama, yak…get it?!)

Disgusted by their lack of vision…or was it laziness, I starting to pitch the rocks from the field onto the path myself. The students were eventually either shamed or motivated into dropping their regular chores for a few hours every day and pitched in. They worked with me on the road until it was finished. Even the monks joined in at some point, over the protests of the students who did not think it was fitting work for these holy wisemen.

I did not know for sure when I started to build that road that it could not fail. That muddy trail packed with stones and tractorloads of grainy sand and clay was destined to become a strong, solid road, a fitting pathway to the Lamas. We built a road that withstood not only the torrential winter rains soon to be upon us, but one that remained unchanged to this day of writing, twenty years and thousands of pairs of feet later.

My heart suffered though, building that road. The weather turned colder, and suddenly my architect was distracted. He became inordinately interested in helping finish the walkway instead of working on his drawings. The reason was not hard to find.

The stunningly beautiful Caroleen had returned to the Tibetan Centre to spend time with the monks and help prepare their house for the winter. Last year she had broken a young student's heart, devastated him. She would eat up my naive little architect and spit out the pieces.

To see them working side by side in the drizzling rain made my blood boil and my stomach churn…Passion in the country has its moments. My mind asked endless tortured and unanswerable questions… "Did she have to be such a good worker as well as being beautiful? Did he have to give her his raincoat while he toiled beside her drenched and shivering? Did she have to look so damn good soaking wet?… I must get him back, I must protect him."

I fantasized, I prayed, I suffered and plotted, finally devising a sinister plan to gain back his full attention. I began having fainting spells, murmuring softly, "It's nothing", when I came reluctantly back to life. I sighed, I stared into space, I let it be known very gently that I had an incurable illness… one day at lunch actually falling completely out of a chair onto the parquet floor where I lay unrevivable for a good five minutes. The perfect Drama Queen.

The plan was working well, my architect buzzed around attentively, and Caroleen's attention was turned to the next victim. It was a tense time when my Father and stepmother returned from

Hawaii. I begged the architect not to worry them by telling of my "illness," but once into the lie, how to get out?

When father announced one evening that the American lady Lorraine would be joining us for dinner, I thought nothing of it.

A dining room is perhaps an unusual place for a small, personal miracle to occur, however this was no ordinary dining room. We sat at a twenty-foot long table of dark oak, medieval size, with massive curled table legs holding the weight of the four-inch thick tabletop as if it were just a wisp of chiffon. Family and friends sitting down to dinner, only the roaring fire to keep us warm in an otherwise wintercold castle.

Our Spanish highback carved leather armchairs were pieces of art, the brass studs reflecting the dancing firelight. The surrounding walls of huge square cut stones were golden honey and sand in color, grayed slightly here and there by five hundred years of age. The *pisé* floors of this beautiful room had been restored meticulously by local craftsmen to the original design. Perfect to the last smooth circle of river stones set in ever widening arcs to form a medieval mosaic that was somehow warm to little bare feet. A safe place to be, a solid place to be, this family room of Chateau de Chaban.

Although there is a formal dining room upstairs, this huge downstairs kitchen was always the heart of the castle. Located at the base of the central stone spiral staircase, it was the crossroads of our lives. Four doors led to different parts of those lives. One took us to the working kitchen where food was prepared. From that room a smaller door opened onto a hidden wooden staircase to the upper floors, a much needed shortcut to the bedrooms above.

The second door led outside to the western façade and flagstone patio, with its soft view over the gardens and valley. We dined often here in the summer, and winter too in clement weather.

A third door, dark and studded with nails, led to the wine cellar, with its treacherous *oubliette* dropoff hidden behind the opened door.

The fourth door opened onto the huge stone staircase, the backbone of the castle. It wound up five stories to the very top of the tallest tower, past the main dining room, past the library and guest room with its four poster bed, and past the round astrology room with the pieshaped bed father designed to fit its beautiful contours without blocking the small stone fireplace.

The ascending staircase narrows, spiraling tighter and tighter, then suddenly you are out in the open sky. No door at the very top, just a step-through opening onto the best view in the world. A small round tower, open to the sun, stars, moon and all the elements. In ancient times guards were stationed at this watchtower to survey the surrounding land for miles in all directions. Even with the countryside so peaceful, so balmy, the scenario is easy to imagine; you can almost hear the faintest clanking of armor, the neighing of restless horses, the scuffle of boots on stone.

Now, in this century of high tech warfare, the open tower nestling above the tallest trees is infinitely better suited for picnics, graceful exercising, soulful meditation, or plain old stargazing.

Descending the flight of endless stone steps, one hundred or so in all, inspires different age groups in varying ways. The youngest make their way carefully, clinging to the wrought iron railing that follows the outer arc of the wall; teenagers race down without missing a beat; old folks tread sedately, also balancing on the railing. My father always ran. Up or down, always in a hurry to get started on the next project or thought, the stairs only the means to reach his destination.

I on the other hand, preferred dawdling… stopping at each window to peer through the intricate stained glass windows, many dated in the sixteenth century as I noticed on a recent visit.

Each colorful scene looks out over a different vista. Each view is slightly distorted through the uneven handmade glass, thus the bright yellow of a unicorn or the black and royal blue of a prince in armor offers a unique, kaleidoscope landscape.

Every landing displayed a beautiful carved wooden door to one of those wondrous huge rooms. Finally reaching the bottom landing and the last door, I would be enveloped by the warm air of the meeting place, the intersection, the kitchen, where deep soft armchairs faced the crackling flames in the fireplace on every winter day of the year. Without a doubt the busiest room in the castle, this was a boisterous, busy, comfy, place, where meals were rarely taken with less than ten people seated at the grand old table.

Tonight, Father and Maritee's friend Lorraine, a gifted translator of large intellectual and political Spanish tomes, has joined us for dinner. This was the first time I had met Lorraine. She seemed perfectly charming, despite whisperings one heard about her odd behavior.

It was into this cozy space, with its laughter and clink of glasses and silverware that a new and strange energy appeared. In the middle of the meal, and for no apparent reason, Lorraine suddenly began rocking back and forth…going on about colors so brilliant she couldn't describe them, using words I couldn't understand.

Being a practical, recently transplanted California girl who knows a wacko when she sees one, I immediately moved the child sitting next to her, one of my little stepsisters, over to my right side, leaving Lorraine sitting on my left, the space of the missing child between us.

A tension filled the room that rivaled the immeasurable power of a lion crouched to spring; the quivering skin, thrashing tail, wickedly lolling tongue, the intensity of the eyes, the surging liftoff. Through these five foot thick stone castle walls, came the proverbial dense air you could "cut with a knife."

Chaos I couldn't pin down was happening all around. Father had tears rolling down his cheeks, sitting across the huge dark oak table from Lorraine; he was saying something that sounded like. "It's all right, let it happen, we are friends here."

The rocking and gibberish intensified, then suddenly turning directly to me and looking into my cynical eyes, Lorraine said "Bernadette, I have a message for you."

I said nothing… too astonished to speak, but thought very loudly, "What! With all these people here!?"

As if my thoughts were shouted out loud, every other person in the room mysteriously melted away.

While Lorraine stared at me with wild, piercing eyes, my stepmother rounded up her three daughters and left the room. I remember thinking, "It's none too soon, they should not be seeing this crazy person carry on like this."

The beautiful blue eyed young angel of an architect with whom I was having that extraordinary affair, got up and left the room. I say extraordinary because of his incredible gentleness and kindness. This airy fairy waif butted against my aggressive California ways with silence and a smile on his lips that made my heart melt. At this moment, I was relieved to see him go.

My father also got up, just up and left the table on a mysterious errand… and I was alone, alone with Lorraine and The Energy. Why would they all leave the room when something interesting or crazy was about to happen?

Still now, no longer rocking, Lorraine put her face close to mine and said, "*You have got to stop what you are doing, it is dimming the light in your eyes.*"

Now any fool knows the eyes are the Windows of the Soul, even a California girl, and I thought myself nobody's fool. But in the face of this blatant challenge, (and I knew exactly what stupid and now apparently dangerous thing the message was referring to), my only thought was one of curiosity…

Who *up there* could be watching me so closely? What else were they seeing? Who had 'passed on' that was close enough to me to care? My father's mother was dead, but I had not been close to her, didn't even like her very much. Those thoughts flashed through my mind at warp speed.

The thought of my lost little brother Christopher never crossed my mind. He had been a tot when he left us and that is how I would always remember him… this was adult stuff. "Who could it be?" Reading my thoughts again Lorraine replied,

"This message is not from any one person dear."

As my brain still dealt with the practical aspect of *who* could be spying on me from up there, and why didn't they mind their own business, Lorraine lifted a necklace over her head and placed it over mine, saying only, "This will protect you."

Like magic, all the characters from the earlier scene - my father, stepmother, three children and my architect, came back into the dining room in little groups, sat down and resumed eating as if they had never left. Lorraine carried on perfectly normally and everyone had a lovely evening, everyone that is except me…what on earth was going on?

Going to Lorraine's room upstairs later, I asked her what had happened. She replied with a worried frown, "Why dear, what did I do?"

"You gave me a message," I said, "Who was it from?" Closing her eyes quietly for a moment, she said the words I had never heard before, this being twenty or so years ago, words imprinted on my mind like it happened today, words that I now hear used with casual frequency. "It was not from any one person dear, it was from the Universal Consciousness."

The cynic in me did not allow any feelings of awe, gratitude or need for immediate change. Puzzlement, yes. I called my sister Jenny in Switzerland, that lovely, funny, beautiful person who is close to a saint in my eyes, for she can always manage to "keep her head when all about are losing theirs."

I related what had happened, and asked her, "Why would anyone up there want to help me?" She listened intently, never asking what stupid or dreadful thing I had been doing to inspire this gift of a special message. She simply said when I was finished, *"Don't ask why, just say Thank You and go on."*

I have been thanking God ever since.

Although mystified at the time, I was still too stubborn to take the message at face value and stop my 'illness' farce immediately. Within the next two weeks or so however, I no longer felt the need to perpetuate the dangerous train of thought that was harmful to no one except me, *and the light in my eyes.*

* * * * *

Surrounded by mystics and monks, is it any wonder we led a charmed life. While Lorraine's strange psychic gift was kept a hushed secret and her privacy protected, the Lamas on the other hand welcomed visitors. People came from miles around to see them, to be in their presence if only for a few brief minutes; and even the most skeptical persons left the meeting with new respect, and a thoughtful, calm demeanor.

Although never a direct student of the Lama's teachings, I admired their ability to hang onto their serenity in a land of relative chaos compared to the orderly ways of their lost monasteries, and have witnessed first hand several powerful displays of healing.

A few years after Lama Gendun came to live in the Dordogne, he saved my little sister's life. Child number eight in the chronological order of things, Alexandra was Father's first child with his second wife, Maritee, my ex roommate. The pony the child was riding on became rambunctious and dumped her off at full speed… she struck her head on a rock and was knocked unconscious.

Picking up the limp little body and shouting for someone to fetch Lama Gendun, Father carried the child up the outside staircase of the thirteenth century stone tower that lead to his immense bedroom in the western wing of the castle. Inside the room, suspended above the gleaming parquet floors, hung a giant swinging bed… a heavy oak frame supporting the lightest of fluffy down comforters. Thick chains hooked in the massive overhead beams stretched down to fasten at each corner of the bed.

Father gently lay the child on the comforter, a tiny, lifeless Sleeping Beauty. Unlike the first batch of seven California transplants, this sweet little eight year old was one hundred percent 'made in France', with the prettiest little accent when speaking English you would ever hope to hear. We all wanted very much to hear that pretty voice.

Turning her over on her side gently so her mother and I could look at the wound, we saw surprisingly, not a lot of blood, but a gaping hole at the base of the skull where it joined the neck. A hole I looked into myself, and could have put my baby finger into.

Knowing enough not to breath germs into the injury, we stood back and waited and prayed, yes, prayed Christian prayers.

Lama Gendun came up the ancient stairway in a rush, threw open the heavy wooden door as if it were a toy, and began waving his arms in the air, talking and chanting, clearing the air of any negative powers.

He leaned over the child, saw where the hair was parted and the deep hole in all its vulnerability was exposed to the world, and did something that would make modern doctors quail…he blew a tremendous garlicky breath directly onto the opening.

Saying only, "She will be alright, but I would like you to call the French doctor to see her and take X-rays if needed." He exited the room with a smile and a nod to all. The little girl half stirred and smiled, we looked at the wound again, and I swear to you *there was a film of matter over the hole.*

The French doctor arrived soon thereafter, examined the now cheerful child, and said in a show of respect that we were becoming accustomed to, "We will take X-rays tomorrow after she has rested, but my feeling is if Lama Gendun says she is alright, then she is alright."

No X-rays were ever taken, the wound was only a small speck the next day, and the child so full of energy, Maritee had to remind her to take it easy for the next few days.

THE LORD'S PRAYER

As I write, I see a man in flowing robes sitting crosslegged on a beach, facing the sea, humming and communing with nature. I approach him quietly in my mind's eye, and see it is not a Tibetan monk, but "J.R." of Dallas fame, sitting on the beach in Malibu.

Before that stretch of beach and quiet bay became inundated with celebrities, back when it was my playground and my world, Larry Hagman was one of the few actors in residence that I recognized. We kids used to giggle and point at him then, sitting so still and off in his own world, but it appears he knew something we didn't, as anyone who meditates, exercises, or benefits from breathing exercises will now tell you.

For myself, with a constantly dancing Gemini mind, I find meditation a bit long to get into, and prefer a double whammy of the Lord's Prayer. Not in its original state mind you… I like to think my sister wrote my epitaph when she said in admiration one day, seated in a flowering garden in France I had wrought out of stony land, "Bernadette, you always leave everything better than it was."

Perhaps you will not agree, and find I have gone too far by rewriting a small portion of The Lord's Prayer.

The phrase *"Lead us not into temptation"* never sat well with me. Is it conceivable I wondered, that God would purposely 'lead us' into temptation? I think not, and prefer a 'translation glitch' theory.

After deliberation at the oddest moments on the subject, it came to me as a flash, one of those ideas that seem to fly into your head without any prior thought or provocation; and it felt right. That phrase which used to catch in my craw so badly "Lead us not into temptation", I would now recite happily as, "*let us not yield* to temptation." What do you think?

My first recitation of the Lord's Prayer is radial, flowing over family and friends, then out to anyone in need… radiating as far as the Rain Forests and their disappearing inhabitants, although I sometimes wonder about the effectiveness of this due to the dissipation factor.

The second recitation is very specific. "Thank You for everything that is going right, God. Please take care of the continued health and happiness of my daughter and myself," and then a clear focus on my current goals.

I attribute my survival and mild successes to these conversations with God. So why don't I pray more often given the success rate? I equate it lightly to my foolishness regarding taking the vitamins that make me feel better…as soon as I feel better, I forget to take the vitamins.

I have been happy with this version of the Lord's Prayer for many years, yet as I commit these thoughts to paper, convinced that God would not set out to trap us, to tempt us, I can't help but see Adam and Eve in the Garden of Eden; the tricky snake begins *hiss sultry flirting*; the first salesman, *out to sell hiss first apple…* or was it a pomegranate.

I need help on this one… if Adam and Eve had rejected the apple, and Paradise was not lost, then in this age of precarious job security, would God still have a job?

Why does this story portray God tempting the Keepers of the Garden, knowing the outcome yet proceeding with the setup? Who started this Adam and Eve story, and why does it get so much play? Someone please tell me this is not something I need to lose sleep over.

Reading these last few paragraphs later in a 'rewrite' phase, I trip over my own question; 'Is there a possibility God was indeed tempting Adam and Eve with the luscious apple?' Now I am sure of my answer… abashed that I thought otherwise or had more than a fleeting moment of doubt.

No one tempts me but myself. We have our free will; the Choice is always ours, the responsibility always ours… every decision is an opportunity to see who we want to be, what we are made of, what we want out of life.

There are higher choices, and not so high choices; the apple may represent the latter. I don't pretend to know why, a guess would be so there was relativity, something to get the ball rolling in the realm of choice… a game perhaps.

I want to run and look for my cherub now, my heart is pulling me out the door. It is pitch black outside, no moon tonight, I stop on the porch for a think… do I really want to go stumbling around in the dark, up and down the lanes to her various friends asking her whereabouts? I think not. No, I'll wait the last half hour, give her a chance to surprise me, see if she shows up at ten, her regular curfew.

I will write a few more pages, and pray she will be home by ten, thus sparing me the grief of searching for her in the dark. Interrogating neighbors and friends as to her whereabouts is just the beginning… then the impossible task of dragging her unwilling body home if she doesn't want to come.

Any humiliation another might find in this prospect has long since ceased to work its wiles on me; probably since the day years ago when I rifled through my first real love's top dresser drawer in his Beverly Hills home, spurred on by that infallible woman's intuition that we are blessed, or cursed with.

Around my neck was the sweet gold necklace John had given me for Christmas, the one with my initials grandly etched on the face, and something tender I don't remember on the back. Carefully probing the occupants of the drawer, my guilty, searching fingers touched a box. Opening it with a sick trepidation, my worst fears (for that young stage of my life) were confirmed. In the box lay not one, not two, nor three identical necklaces, but five. Only the initials were different.

Where does the stomach go when it drops? What causes that physical blow that knocks the wind out of you and forces you to sit before you fall? Is it the shattering of your dreams? Is it the loss of trust in this person you wanted so much to believe in? Is it fear crashing into your psyche, nestling there like a viper, in the void left after innocent love has been booted out… mutating insidiously into unconscious suspicion of every man who enters your life in the future.

John tracked me down at the castle ten years later and asked me to meet him in Paris for a weekend. Stunned and curious, I agreed. This bad boy is attractive, funny, entertaining, and born rich, a Ferrari in his mouth instead of the proverbial silver spoon. Most of his time since then has been spent trying to divest of his fortune with a variety of precarious adventures.

By his telling, he was the only American entry in the Paris to Dakar race two years in a row, something that presumably is verifiable if one were interested. His co-pilot was a girl not picked for her driving or navigational skills, but her lovely companionship.

Halfway through the strenuous course, their vehicle off-course and broken down, they had to spend the night in a tent. When the tinkling of small bells woke the lady, John professed to hear nothing and went back to sleep. He should not have been so astounded therefore to wake up and find their vehicle had been stripped of every movable part, seats included… carried off silently into the night on the backs of camels, per the tracks that willingly gave up their clues. The tinkling bells were not an imagined friend of Peter Pan's, but an integral if whimsical part of the Bedouin's camel harnesses.

Stilling my skeptical heart, we met on a Friday afternoon in Paris at the Intercontinental Hotel. Two romantic evenings later, in the middle of the night on Saturday, he asked me to marry him. Thrilled but wary I said nothing that I remember, and dozed off to sleep. In the morning, I do remember saying, "I had a dream last night" to which he replied, "It was not a dream, I want you to marry me, I'll send you a ticket, come to Califonia."

Not really believing it, yet not disbelieving it either, I mean, how could someone say that and not mean it, right? I went back to Chaban and told my father… who was *thrilled!* It hadn't occurred to me until that moment when I saw his excitement that he must have been wondering if I was ever going to marry. Being a man, he never asked, and of course Mom wasn't there to bug me, so I probably didn't think of it much myself, if it at all.

John went back to California, the ticket arrived and I started to believe. I was happy, excited, a bit fearful, but ready to take the leap.

Packed in fact, when the telegram arrived. "Slight hold up, don't come this week, Love John."

I didn't hear from him again for another fifteen years... when he called and said he was coming to the Bahamas to see me.

It was surreal. Genevieve and I met him in Marsh Harbour, and returned together to Hopetown by boat. Hotels were full so he gratefully accepted the couch I offered him, and it was as if we had been seeing each other regularly for the past fifteen years... he was still funny and entertaining, he still adored me, and I still amused him. The only difference was we were now both divorced, and each custodian of our only child. I withheld the pieces of the heart he had broken twice in twenty years, determined only to enjoy him as a friend.

He regaled me with stories. It is highly possible this one originated with him as he tells it, and just as likely he borrowed it from someone else. Either way, I wish it had happened to me...

Flying to Paris to spend New Years with a girlfriend on the spur of the moment, he telephoned that wonderful restaurant Maxim's (yes the one just around the corner from my old office in Paris) to make a reservation for dinner one New Year's Eve. The Maitre D' laughed and said "Monsieur, we have been booked for weeks!"

Corky (John's nickname, to thrill him if this is true, to embarrass and annoy him if it is not), tried various persuasions that had worked in the past, to no avail. The last words the maitre D' had for him were, "Je regrette Monsieur, I am very sorry, we do not have a table for you". That was his undoing...

Corky had a beautiful antique table delivered to Maxim's the next morning, then called the Maitre D' that afternoon to see if it had arrived. The Maitre D' was in high good humor… "I give up Monsieur, we will have Your Table ready for you."

Not only was it ready, it was magnificently adorned and placed in the very best location near the center of the dance floor, softly illuminated by a discreet spotlight that transformed it into the centerpiece of Maxim's stunning décor. He will swear this is a true Corky story…I am not so sure, but I love it anyway.

At the end of a weekend of laughter and catching up on twenty years of adventures, he said we had to get together for a long weekend soon, to pick a place, any place, any country I chose, and he would arrange it. Then he hugged me, told me he adored me, and left for California. He called me from there, he called again from Paris, to say Hi and remind me to set up the rendezvous.

I have a life now, I don't leave my daughter at the drop of the hat for anyone, and I needed to know there was a possibility he was serious before I unleashed my enthusiasm again. I suggested *he* set things up then let me know where to meet him. Can you guess? I have still to hear from the little devil. Perhaps in another twenty years when I am waving my cane we will meet again and he will still adore me.

SOUTH AFRICA

A few summers before I met Gen's Dad in the Bahamas, I drove from Paris to the Dordogne for a visit. The Tibetan Center had been progressively undergoing many changes; new buildings, a reception office, a large outdoor kitchen, many more individual meditation A-frame houses scattered about under the trees… only my beautiful, golden lane from the road to the courtyard steps remained unchanged, flat and solid as we had built it. Things were in full swing at the Center, with teachings, seminars, and the promise of a ceremony performed rarely in the Western world, and known simply to us as 'The Black Hat Ceremony'. A high ranking lama had traveled to the Center via Paris to perform this sacred, and particularly powerful ritual.

It is a woeful admission to make, but I remember very little of the actual proceedings, only the power of the positive energy created that day between one heavyset Eastern man sitting on a platform a few feet above the ground, wearing a symbolic black hat of Tibetan origin… and hundreds of Western believers seated at his feet in a huge tent.

At the culminating moment of the Ceremony when the Black Hat is raised off the lama's head and held up for all to see, each person is absorbed by their own different insights, whether it be of peace, healing, love, or something indescribable.

It was at this ceremony I met a wonderful couple from South Africa who were staying at the Center for a month. We became good friends, and when they invited me to visit them in Johannesburg the following summer, I accepted with pleasure.

I took in as much as I could in the few months that I lived with them, and definitely overstayed their kind hospitality. South Africa and its neighbors are far too magnificent to capture in a few pages, but I can try to give a taste to those who have not been there.

Rhodesia, as it was called before becoming Zimbabwe, Kariba Bay, Victoria Falls…these are places mystical and magical. The falls are my favorite. Breathtaking. Crashing froth pours over the edge of the cliffs, mist rises up to spray the foliage along the footpath at the top, watering the orchids, the ferns, the flowers and you.

The falls were also in the middle of the Zambia/Rhodesia border war. From the porch of the Victoria Hotel situated on the Rhodesian side, looking across the Zambezi River to the Zambia riverbank, you could see armed soldiers lurking in the bushes below… hopefully guided by a mandate not to shoot stupid tourists, or where would the money come from to support their ongoing wars?

Soldiers guarding the splendid old colonial hotel walked around with rifles casually on their shoulders or sloppily under their arms. Following a "rifle under the arm" guard up the sweeping staircase, I found the business end of the rifle a few inches from my face. One had to be more careful of the guards, loose from good living at the hotel, than of the enemy; not that I could tell which was which even if I had stumbled over them

Kariba Bay, I saw my first wild hippo, lumbering along a small lane at night intent on regaining his waterhole. He passed by the car window close enough for me to touch his back, which was in fact as tall as the top of the car door. But I had heard hippos are one of the most dangerous animals in the wild, their sudden speed and crushing jaws belied by their great weight and apparent lack of attention to what is going on around them… and I sat on my hands.

Traveling with friends from Johannesburg to the Republic of Congo, it seemed like being in a video war game to arrive at the Kinshasa airport and be herded immediately into a convoy of trucks and buses. The local military was determined to keep these valuable tourists from harm.

Thus from our perch on the front seat of a comfortable small bus, we were facing the back end of the truck in front of us… with a *cannon* mounted on its flatbed, trained just above our heads. Until then it hadn't really clicked that we were in a war zone. It soon became all too clear however that we were on unfamiliar and dangerous turf. Being escorted to a photo safari camp in an *anti-mine vehicle*, we were told that this was a version of Hummer constructed specifically for this part of the world… so that the front cabin, along with its passengers, would break off and roll away from the remainder of the vehicle upon hitting an exploding mine.

As this was being explained in great detail, I did wonder for a brief moment if we had picked a good time to go traipsing around Africa. Two weeks after we left Kinshasa airport, two commercial planes were shot down, killing 52 tourists

Not to be deterred by a the local wars, we went anywhere we could that was a hop away by private puddlejumper, those little five-seater planes that are able to take off and land on mere patches of dirt runway.

Traveling by the small local airlines was also an eye opener. While we checked in duffle bags, most of the other passengers were tossing rifles on the ticket counter, for which they received a baggage claim check. The counter looked like an arsenal. Somehow these weapons found their way back to their rightful owners at the other end of the trip, and I felt rather left out, not having a rifle or a pistol to claim.

My softest, kindest image in this country of wild contradictions is of a golf course at sunset, scattered with dainty springboks grazing or laying in the shade trees at the fringes of the course. Magnificent secretary birds strolled unperturbed across the greens, the last of the golfers waiting patiently for them to go about their secretary bird business.

I have been blessed with sights of red elephants. Red from playing in a dusty claybowl, stomping happily around in the swirling red stuff like mischievous kids, large kids. A huge bull stands apart from the herd at the edge of the nearby waterhole, swinging his head back and forth, contemplating the murky water, deciding whether it is too late for a bath.

Walking along the small trail back to camp late the next afternoon, a sight forty yards away stops me in my tracks. The same lone bull elephant from yesterday calls out to my camera. On the opposite bank of the watering hole, he is by himself today. Kneeling down with a thump, he rolls back and forth in the dust until he has covered every inch of himself in the red, red clay.

Getting to his feet, quite gracefully given the massive tonnage, he lifts his trunk, then freezes; a giant redbronze statue glinting in the rays of the setting sun, huge tusks aloft in the air, trunk reaching to the sky. A red elephant in a red sunset, and me with no film. The raised trunk trembles; I fear my red statue may be sniffing me out, and back quietly into the underbrush.

A quiver of the ears, a huge shake of that colossal body and the bull disappears in a billowing red cloud…to reappear a few breathless seconds later, now magically dressed in his everyday gray suit… the perfect trick. A missed Kodak moment that trumpets vividly from the top drawer of my mind's golden jewelbox.

I do have photos of baby zebra with stripes so fine and distinct, that Picasso himself would be tempted to leave them thus in their perfection. Two baby lions sunning sleepily on a huge gray boulder, peek lazily over the top at me to see if any mischief is in the making… their mother very likely much nearer than I knew as I snapped their portrait.

The most dramatic photo I took in Africa shows me face to face with death. A magnificent male lion, this regal patriarch takes up the entire frame of my camera. Crouched to spring, his mouth is open, red tongue flicking sideways in anticipation of lunch, his eyes are glaring into mine, black pupils a fierce dot in the golden orbs… suddenly a frantic tug on my arm conveys I am much too close. Still clicking, I back away and turn quickly to jump in the waiting vehicle, amidst angry admonitions from my friends that I should be more careful.

I did not realize what they were talking about until the photos were developed. I am so ready to be that lion's lunch.

.

From Johannesburg it is a fairly quick hop by plane to the Isles of Mauritius and Reunion, home at the time to two truly exotic Club Meds. A young honeymoon couple at one of these resorts became an unexpected casualty of the Club's reputation for fun in the sun. Shocked and embarrassed, the young husband watched his new bride became truly intoxicated with the erotica of the Islands, or perhaps it was the abundant wines. Throwing her inhibitions and clothes to the winds, she became suddenly addicted to frolicking naked in the sea with whoever was interested in joining her. Sharing his wife's breasts, and other body parts so recently acquired, was not on this groom's agenda, and brokenhearted, he headed for home... alone.

Nearby are the Seychelle Islands, jewels of the Indian Ocean. Take the best weather of the Bahamas, add its lush flora and abundant sealife, paint in misty mountains, wild forests, and tea plantations; create the most spectacular, clear, sharp light for photography I have seen anywhere in the world, and you have the Seychelles.

It was here that I came this close to being molested by a giant octopus. Snorkeling lazily back to the beach from a wondrous reef full of swirling, flashing, friendly tropical fish as curious about me as I was amused by their antics, I headed slowly towards the shore. Swimming face down across a shallow sandy area in about five feet of water, a large mass of speckled yellow sand glided towards me, moving fast.

Before I could put on the brakes, a solid wall of color shot up two feet from my face, a psychedelic pinwheel four feet across, pulsing with color and energy, transforming from golds, browns and blacks to vivid pinks and oranges... moving shades of spots and ripples, a glowing spinning wheel...and what's this? Tentacles? Long, sucky tentacles appearing at the outskirts of the glorious spinning wheel.

The spinning stopped, and I was gifted with an intense display of power, energy, and pride in the pulsing colors as we faced each other, eye to eye in that suspended moment of time.

Reaching out one strong, sticky tentacle, the octopus gingerly fondled my reflecting mask and snorkel. I quivered, desperate to flee yet not daring to move. Deciding we were not sexually compatible, the huge sea creature suddenly folded down his power play, became a horizontal, gliding mass once more, and raced off with a wicked gleam in his roving eye. I began to breathe again, and humbly floated in on the waves to the silky beach, stunned with rapture and the aftershock of my explosive underwater encounter.

Crossing in a daze over the little spit of sand to a fresh water lagoon formed at the base of a crystal cascade falling from above, I sank into its cool embrace. Protected from lusting octopi by the familiar lush ferns and tropical fronds waving in the breeze, I lay on my back, gazed at the brilliant blue sky, and just floated.

I could have stayed forever in this wondrous part of the world, but after eight months I thought I had rather overstayed my welcome. The original invitation had been on the order of, "Oh do come and visit", and although my hosts still appeared happy to see me, I knew it was time to go.

My lovely South African friends, I have lost touch with you. Should you ever read this, please, "Do come and visit" for as long as you like.

From South Africa I returned to France and Chaban, always my base, now my sanctuary. I had several more adventures in the south of France with a terribly handsome and conniving French American who really does not deserve space in these pages, although his way of life was perhaps even more outrageous than what we have sped through so far. Perhaps another time.

When I refused to be part of this mad man's shenanigans any longer, Jean Pierre introduced me to his friend in Paris, the American lawyer I lived with for two years before moving to Nassau. In Nassau I met the Marlboro Man, and the rest is history.

My pretty girl is still not home, ten minutes to go before I throw in the towel and track her down… No getting around it, I am really missing her now, it's very hard to stay put and wait for her. At the stroke of 10p.m. I will go and find her… time to write a few more lines….

THE HOPETOWN LIGHTHOUSE

The weather here in the Abacos during the 'winter' months is something to thank God for. For those of you in cold, dreary or wet winter circumstances, I don't know if a description of a winter day here would make you angry, or weepy with desire, but I will try to capture the beauty of it for you.

The pounding of the Atlantic surf is muffled in the northern distance behind me. Directly in front of me, the Sea of Abaco ripples quietly beneath our porch. The cottage is poised on a slight rocky raise on the harbor side of the thin finger of land separating the two seas…no more than a spit of 200 yards of sand and rock upon which we perch rather precariously.

Dancing ripples of color flow from the wakes of busy boats heading out of the harbor to begin their day. Motorboats, sailboats, trawlers, ferries, yachts, and sleek private seaplanes…the wake-ripples all begin alike, a dark, dark blue swell in the deep water of the channel, dissolving into emerald and turquoise miniwaves washing over the sandbar and into the shallows.

Ultimately, and in their own good time, those same ripples reach our porch all molten silver and gold, reflections from the perfect sand just inches below. The sun shines, the birds sing, and life is unusually close to perfect.

Threatening waves from the outside world are subdued by the lazy curves of the land as it forms one of the world's most picturesque small harbors.

Circled by colorful pastel cottages sitting on patchwork bits of land that no one wants to sell, the sailboats bob serenely on their moorings and yachts nestle up to their docks. Our cottage faces southwest, where the sunsets over the candy striped lighthouse are worth stopping whatever you are doing to catch the show; a blaze of orange and silver, a blast of red, a darkening of the sky and you think it's over.

Suddenly, for those in the know and still watching, there is a last minute flash, a glow of lavender, pink and fuchsia that lights up the clouds, the sky, the lighthouse; another Kodak moment, if you have your camera ready.

The red and white striped lighthouse of Hopetown is famous. As of this writing it is one of the few remaining in the world still operated manually and fueled by kerosene. It basks in the admiration of all by day. By night it returns the favor, sending warm rays softly over the town's sleeping residents. A stronger, clearer beam goes out to tired sea travelers, guiding them home, or safely on their way to other destinations.

One hundred steps to the top of the lighthouse, and a 360 degree view that will take your breath away.

On my porch a cloud crosses the sun, a dark menacing cloud. I am suddenly reminded less of the beautiful days, but rather the stormy nights I have encountered here. "*Son et lumiere*" nights; when Sound and Light shows rip the sky with millions of megawatts of electricity, blinding flashes lighting the entire contour of the mouth of the harbor and Eagle Rock island.

By day Eagle Rock is a pretty scene, with its empty house and overturned boat that is never used. By stormy night it becomes a perfect movie set for a haunted house. Bursts of lightning shoot jaggedly up from the waterline to heaven, the windows and doors of the house are now the eyes and mouth of an eerie monster. Thunder and drum rolls accompany this fiesta of the gods, and I am but a naïve witness to the powers of Nature.

Thoughts of Gen are flooding my mind now, a recent silly 'gardening' episode has filled me with a warmth I want to share with her.

Bicycling to the edge of town one morning I spied blossoms of 'Four O'clocks' under the trees in vibrant colors I had not seen before. They called out to me. I got off the bike to say hello. Deep purples, brilliant whites splashed with fuchsia. Miniature paintings made by a wildly creative artist, they peeked timidly out from under a pile of rubble a careless gardener must have dumped upon them.

Getting out the long tuberous bulb was harder than I thought, and I returned to the cottage for a trowel. Returning to the scene thus armed, Genevieve has reluctantly been talked into helping me. Acting more as "lookout" than gardener, she does very little digging, and lots of giggling. Issuing frantic orders for me to "Stop!" every five minutes, she pretends we are just chatting as friends approach on bikes and golfcarts. I can only resume digging when they have passed, the coast is clear, and the waving and salutations are over.

Despite the constant interruptions, in half an hour we have enough plants to insure the continuation of the species. A bag of treasures on the handlebar of each bike, we head for home. Transplanted to a semi-shaded corner of my garden, the uprooted plants sulk and droop. For three days they hang their heads in shock and distress, wilted and miserable… I know exactly how they feel.

Miraculously the fourth day they come back to the living, raise their little heads and begin to look around. They like this place, they like the extra attention and plentiful water. The shade is good, the sun is just right. As one, they decide this is a good place to be. Sending a signal to their roots to "unfurl and dig in", they reward us a few days later with a profusion of splashy blooms, exquisite trumpet shapes not much bigger than my thumb. Gen and I stare and smile, it is a lovely moment.

This is when I am at my happiest, nurturing my flowers and my child, watching them grow, watching them bloom. I am so thankful to have the time to appreciate these things now… the serenity of it, the peace of mind.

So it is puzzling that now that our life together is so good, now that I have no deadlines, no crises to deal with, really very little to do at all except enjoy myself and get my daughter off to school in the morning… why then, after I wave to Gen as she passes in front of the cottage on the school ferry, are there days that I crash back into bed, unable to move or even get up to eat?

I sleep the sleep of the dead, getting up barely in time to put on a cheerful face and cook something hot for my girl, who arrives home from school at four o'clock, ravenous.

In Nassau, I took this same lethargy to be an offshoot of emotional upheaval, unresolved problems, and running the Restaurant alone and nonstop for too long. I thought it must stem from being exhausted on a daily basis, to the point of not knowing how I drove to the Restaurant every morning and again every evening… did not see other cars or pedestrians until the last minute; was on remote control 80% of the time, eyes fighting to close. A miracle I didn't kill myself or others.

Moving to Hopetown, has been a revelation. For the first time in years, I have time to think, to regroup, to write. The computer facing my window on the world beckons, and on 'good days' I am able to produce interesting pages. With Genevieve content in our surroundings, I now have time to assess this zombielike state I still find myself struggling with despite our newfound happiness. In the past it was easy to put the blame on being overworked, burned out, drained from the hell that was Nassau. It seemed logical to think that here in the peace and serenity we had carved out for ourselves, I would soon be put to rights.

So now what was wrong? A bit of gardening is all I can accomplish before resorting to a 'lie down' which can last for hours. Rising reluctantly from blissful slumber minutes before my Gen girl gets home, it's back to the soft down pillows at 9pm, to sleep soundly all night. If eight hours of sleep is enough for most adults, why do I need fourteen?

I thoroughly expected the dragging on my mind and body to release me in this emerald haven, the energy drained from me to be recharged. I counted on the magic of this place to restore my flow of creative ideas, to fill me to bursting with the desire to accomplish a myriad of things.

The reality is quite different. It is a push to rally up enough energy to vacuum the cottage once a week, when I would like to do it daily. Dropping off the laundry a hundred yards down the little lane into town is a major production, and what a feeling of relief when I have a surge of energy that allows me to fix myself a snack to eat.

Time flies by with no apparent change in energy level, My thoughts are ones I have not known for years however; bliss, gratitude, joy. Every day I thank God I don't have to drive to that restaurant again, don't have to deal with the domestic crises of forty staff, don't have to worry about being robbed or my daughter raped. This part of life is grand.

Yet as time continues to flow, a nagging voice begins darting in and out of my mind, now devoid of all pressures, and therefore probably quite empty; *"You should be recovering by now, you should be feeling great, maybe you have one of those unsolvable diseases like Chronic Fatigue"*…a most tedious disease which gives you nothing tangible to hang your hat on, nothing earthshattering to garner sympathy or interest.

Even a liver ailment would be better than that, a residue perhaps of the strange illness that attacked me at age eighteen in France; terrible pains in my kidneys and lower back for weeks before I turned a shade of yellow that couldn't be ignored.

French doctors diagnosed a form of jaundice from tainted seafood. Their experimental treatment consisted of daily injections of embryonic calf's liver, administered by my father's secretary, and instructions not to move from my four-poster bed in the chateau for two months. My mother is nowhere in this memory, perhaps she has already done the Great Split.

To my mind it would be preferable to have confirmation that I am "medically challenged," rather than one of the other options. That I could just be lazy, undisciplined, or depressed is not something I want to admit.

Yet my heart says it can not be depression… I am thrilled by a hummingbird sipping from our feeder, laugh when our fan-tailed pigeon Fred is too lazy to fly around the block; just flaps his wings vigorously and hovers a few inches above the porch railing to get some exercise. I'm happy beyond description when I get an unsolicited hug from my Gen, or see her face glow when she is pleased.

All those times when I thought I must just be lazy, when my life felt like a car running on two cylinders instead of six, perhaps there was another reason. I have to find out. Gen and I don't have that much time left together, she will fly off in a very few years to her own destiny. Perhaps I will be lucky enough to have a daughter who enjoys returning to her mother for visits and chats, but there are no guarantees.

I want to enjoy NOW fully. Want to find out what causes these oh so boring symptoms; fatigue that fourteen hours of sleep does not dispel, lack of appetite, dull mind, odd depth perception at times, achy joints, hips shoulders, neck, chronic congestion, (*if I could breath properly and get oxygen to my poor brain*, I could rule the world!), stabbing pains in my left shoulder when moving too fast in the wrong direction etc. etc.

These are minor annoyances in and of themselves that do not stop me from thanking God every day for my beautiful daughter and our lovely life. He gets a lot of thanks also that the Marina and Restaurant income was parlayed into real estate with good resale value, providing enough for us to live on without my having to work for anyone. At the moment there is no way I could count on being anywhere on a daily basis except in my hammock.

So I wait and watch and think and write, and know that Genevieve and I have been guided to this mystical corner of the world, watched over by the great red and white lighthouse, for many reasons. To learn to live in peace together, to be given the time and inclination to write, and to find a way to either live with or find a cure for the mystery lethargy that has plagued my life.

Could I be getting closer to a breakthrough, hot on the trail of something doctors and nurses have scoffed at during my medical exams in the past? Everyone except the nurse here, Nurse Lettie who takes care of this community of boaters, sports fishers and visiting tourists whenever they are feeling accident prone.

They say timing is everything, and it appears I am finally in the right place at the right time. This island where I have felt more real happiness in a few months than I have in a lifetime, is not as cut off from the world as one would think. Miraculously, an American nurse lives two doors down the lane from me. Nurse Lettie is not only intrigued by my ridiculously low blood pressure, but interested enough to read up on it and search out the latest medical findings, which are very few as of this writing, even on the Internet.

This is not just *a Nurse*, this is the community guardian angel who thinks nothing of jumping in a Navy Seal inflatable at midnight in the middle of a raging storm to accompany the Sea Rescue team to a sailboat in distress. The two young children and wife onboard having kept their wits about them to call for help on the VHF radio.

The rescue boat pounds through the high seas in the pitch dark, bucking and plunging over and through the whipped up waves. The safety jackets, designed to inflate at the contact of water when someone goes overboard, have inflated with the first wave that crashes over the bow. Nurse Lettie and the two other rescuers are wet, cold, yet exhilarated. Aboard a once in a lifetime roller coaster ride many of us would rather not experience.

The sailboat is in sight, thrashing out of control in the wind, a man silhouetted at the bow, bent over the anchor chain. The rescue boat's spotlight picks out the anchor swinging wildly a few feet below the bow. The man's hands are trapped in the chain. As the rescue boat pulls near, there is a sudden vicious upward plunge of the sailboat's bow. The anchor pulls down against the thrust, the chain cuts through the bone of the mangled fingers... the fingers drop overboard in slow motion. The man huddled over the chain watches them fall, as the light from the rescue boat illuminates the silent drama.

The sailboat is tossing about too frantically to be boarded from the rescue vessel. A volunteer rescuer dives overboard and catches the deck on a crashing downswing, heaves himself onboard, and heads the sailboat into calmer waters where Nurse Lettie is able to board, and face the hands now wrapped in towels dripping blood.

As the younger boy sobs quietly, "Daddy is alive, Daddy is alive," the unwrapping begins. Nurse Lettie tells the wife to look away while she takes in the damage... "Is it both hands?" the wife asks quietly.

"I'm afraid so" is the calm reply, "Two fingers gone from one hand, three from the other"...

I permit myself to quote this wife's response in the hopes she will be flattered by my admiration for her bravery and sense of humor in the blackest of scenes, rather than upset by the invasion of her privacy...

"My God I'm so glad he's alive," she said with that wonderful nurse holding the wreck of her husband's hands... and in an aside, so only the nurse can hear, "I guess sex will never be the same!"

FORGIVENESS

I hide away quietly in my cottage, grateful that my time is my own, that I can write and read and amuse myself with daydreaming, or thinking over the options my daughter and I have ahead of us. I forget the limitations, forget I sometimes crawl along on just those two cylinders. Knowing that there is perhaps a Tangible Thing to deal with has given me energy. Accepting that it is ok to rest and not feel guilty when the bottom drops out of my blood pressure, this has given me relief and joy.

Living so quietly here I have become used to being alone, although I do not seem to be lonely, which is quite a different thing. There are no longer twinges of guilt about doing as little as possible, no guilt at all now about swinging in my hammock, catching a few rays of tropical sun between the fronds of the coconut palm above me; just rocking gently, thinking how blessed I am.

Thinking how lucky I am that Nature's gifts still thrill me; that a sunset (and they are of spectacular magnitude in this part of the world) still fills me with awe, that the birds singing and fluttering around our bird feeders make me laugh at their antics, that the profusion of rain lilies erupting after a thunderous storm never ceases to amaze me, and my daughter's face… as it lights up when I make her laugh or she has a funny story to tell me… I thank God for that.

When I am feeling lousy, I slip on the arm cuff of the portable blood pressure monitor I bought for $40. It has more than paid for itself in time and doctor's offices I don't have to visit for this lethargy. When the reading is in the neighborhood of 85/60, nowhere near the normal range of 125/90, I rest. And revel in that luxury.

Still apparently a mystery however, is why the level drops so low, and what can be done about it. Is it hereditary? Is it possible my maternal grandmother, the one who committed suicide in Switzerland perhaps suffered from a similar malady? Might not that have aggravated her illness and unhappiness, making life seem unbearable?

We do know the mysterious sleeping bug was passed from me to Genevieve. It concerned me she was often so tired, sleeping a lot even for a teenager. I worried silently about it. On a hunch we began taking her blood pressure on a regular basis for a few weeks, keeping records of the changes. Thankfully her range is not as low as mine, but low enough to affect her.

I asked doctors in Florida and I asked them in Nassau… "Can low blood pressure possibly be contributing to my general dragginess?" They replied unanimously and adamantly… "No, its fine – it is a good thing to have."

I say to them now… "Well you were wrong…*too low* is NOT good…and thanks for leaving me struggling unnecessarily all these years."

Only one suggestion sounded reasonable… "Try more exercise." Twenty minutes of bicycling however didn't help, instead it knocked me out for hours. I am now a firm believer in W.C. Fields' take on strenuous activity… *"Whenever I feel the urge to exercise, I lie down and wait for it to pass."* So that's what I do, and don't even feel guilty about it.

Ever the optimist, I let myself be tempted to imagine the day when I wake up bursting with energy. This invokes conflicting thoughts; what life would be like with lots of energy, versus, "Don't get your hopes up, a solution might be ages away."

Yet my heart is freer knowing that answers may be soon forthcoming. When the time comes that my pretty girl is ready for a more challenging life, concerts, museums, travel, college, etc… I'll need to be able to keep up with her until she is ready to fly on her own.

With her in mind, I recently purchased a lovely house in Fort Lauderdale, either to move into when we are ready, or sell later and make a bit of profit. I've been going back and forth from the Bahamas to Fort Lauderdale for years, not sure how I find the energy to make these trips, yet they actually seem to give me energy. It is another world to me in Florida; user friendly, clean, green, easy to navigate, packed with a myriad of restaurant choices and unique shops, a people place, and not that far from home. Gen and I both feel very comfortable there.

A hop away from both Nassau and Hopetown, Fort Lauderdale is usually only a 60 minute flight. Taking a book is recommended however; as the airlines find ways to stretch the time anywhere from one to five hours; depending on their disposition, the weather, or planes not always being where they should be at the given time.

The first thing on my Florida list is a drive through Victoria Park, going North along Victoria Park Road from Broward Blvd to Sunrise Blvd. I love the trees, the adjacent water, and particularly the houses on one little cul de sac street along the water. The last time I was there, driving slowly up and down this short little street looking for signs proclaiming a property for sale, I found the perfect house. Three bedrooms, three bathrooms, on a corner lot with a separate downstairs apartment and garage. One of the few two-story houses perched on the little hill with a view past the church, and the boats on the water.

It was for sale by owner, a friendly man I felt immediately comfortable with. He was ready to move up North with his family, and wanted to move soon. The house was priced considerably more than I had in mind and worth every penny.

"I don't want you to be insulted if I make an offer in a range I can afford" I said. He replied, "Go ahead, I won't be insulted."

He wasn't. He accepted my offer, I sold my Nassau house in a flash and at a good profit, and we closed the sale three weeks later.

Then I panicked.

Why did I buy another house? Why didn't I just leave the money from the Nassau house in a bank getting interest? Wouldn't Gen be better off if anything happened to me with some cash rather than a house in Florida?

I spent a week barely able to function, convinced I had made a terrible mistake…it was the first time I had ever heard the expression "buyers remorse," yet now it was being bandied about like a common phrase. A week later the house was leased to tenants per my original plan, the panic retreated, and reason returned. The house could be sold easily and at a profit - if the money had been left in the bank I would have spent it - Gen and I could use the downstairs apartment whenever we were in Fort Lauderdale. Etc.

But the terrible, paralyzing fear I had lived with for a week made me wonder once again, just what was not right with me. And how did I have the energy to buy a large house, when I couldn't find the strength to vacuum the tiny one I lived in?

The mystery is partially solved. I am a very upbeat person with funks, and can now trace the funks with my little machine to that excessively low blood pressure. Which comes first, the chicken or the egg, I do not yet know.

* * * * *

Since Genevieve and I moved to our tranquil, easy place on our little island, she and her Dad talk often on the phone. He is very happy to see her whenever she can get to Nassau, and even the stepmom appears to enjoy spending time with Genevieve, now that there is rarely an opportunity. That is not meant to be bitter, it is just an odd fact of life and a common trait in most of us, to appreciate things once they are gone.

Gen's Dad has even spent a weekend here with her at the cottage in Hopetown, while I went to Ft. Lauderdale to give them some space. The stepmom showed up one day also, accompanying her daughter's class on a field trip. They stopped by the cottage to say hello, and Gen got a big hug from her little sister. The *now* is pretty much ok, it is the *then* I still haven't dealt with.

Forgiveness is a funny thing. As I understand it now from an article in, "On Course, Inspiration for the Inner Journey", by Dr. Michael Ryce, forgiveness *has nothing to do with letting another off the hook for their offenses*. According to Ryce, the root meaning of *forgiveness* in the ancient Aramaic language, is ***to cancel, untie, or let loose***.

Forgiveness is therefore a tool for changing a reality in the mind, thereby releasing stored, destructive energies from within. *It is not something done to, or for others.* It is an internal healing process that changes your own reality; which is not dependent on the behavior of others.

I understand this concept intellectually, and realize it makes good sense that the void left by letting go of deep rooted anger and pain will be replaced with a positive energy that will enhance my life. Yet even understanding this, I find it difficult to let it all go.

I think it must take an act of faith, rather like letting go of a small lifesaving ring to use both hands to clamber into the rescue boat… unable to hang on to both at the same time.

Time, that healer of all things, is helping. That and of course the distance between us now we have moved to Abaco. The hardest part of this intellectual exercise seems to be forgiving myself for getting Gen into this mess by tossing her Dad out without first exhausting all other options, (even if it was only meant to be a short term tossout). I am however, working on it.

What if my sweet girl, she who is usually so quick to forgive…borne of years of necessity and plenty of practice, has finally hit the bottom of the forgiveness barrel? Am I going to be the one to bear the brunt of her first grudge? Me her mum, who has stood by her through the proverbial thick and thin, who has cried with her and comforted her, am I the one to finally make her snap? No, that would be too cruel.

My anger is long gone, nothing but warm thoughts of her fly round in my head, I need a hug. I feel only love for her, a great warmth I want to share. Why is anger needed to bring this transformation about? Can I not learn to tap into the warmth without the crisis?

Clearly I have been offered this time to think, to impress upon myself the need to get things right, before my plans for a cozy relationship are left high and dry in the speeding wake of her transition to the next phase of her life.

Within three years, perhaps less, the choices will be hers; to spend time with Mom or not; to chat with me about college and friends, or not; to share her joys and fears…or not. What I sow now will be reaped very shortly. I must not screw this up.

*****

I will discuss the matter with God, He will show me how to guide this child, this lovely soul, to the place where she can see clearly, at a younger age than I did, that the happiness and successes she wishes for are hers for the asking. Let her discover sooner than I, that place where you thank God for giving you your desires before you receive them; where you commit, without a shred of doubt, to the belief that you deserve what you set your heart on, and that you will soon have it.

Let her find the place where it is OK to envision goals both big and small, whether of financial, spiritual, or emotional nature; where it is OK to dream big dreams, and OK to pray, knowing your prayers for others are as important as the ones for yourself.

In the context of knowing the above, and seeing the trials and tribulations the past has wrought, I must shake my head to clear it of the wish to beat myself with a big stick. Must remind myself that the tortured months and years my daughter and I went through, alone and afraid, could not have been avoided at that point with my limited understanding of God.

Now I know that the choice is ours, it is all out there; a life of plenty, or a life of want; a life of love, or a life of denial. I want to offer this gift to my daughter in a way she will accept it, will believe it, will try it, and see for herself.

A selfish thought really, to wish her to jump right to knowledge and understanding just on my say so, without doing the homework.

To wish her a life brimming with joy; with joy's opposites rarely rearing their smarmy heads. It is for myself I wish this as much as for her. I don't want to struggle again through her struggles.

Does it matter the source of my motivation? I think not, and will guide her by example, will keep her under my Umbrella of Thankfulness. She is an alert young thing, she sees that our lives are truly more blessed recently, God will help her figure it out.

Genevieve has come home. It is one minute to ten. She is full of smiles and hugs, obviously missing me as much as I missed her. The violent outburst of a few hours ago is behind her, the time spent apart fruitful. *By softening my own approach she will also change her reactions, and if one of us is determined to nourish our good points and downsize the ones we are not proud of, we have given ourselves a new beginning.*

I feel already a lightness of spirit moving through me, beginning to banish the pain of her lost childhood. Stepping carefully now to guide her through these next teenage years with love will be a balm for me. Soon now I will throw off this mantle of regret for the happiness she can never recover.

Children are suffering all over the world, and compared to them I know our life is easy. Yet when you have harmed someone you love by your own actions, these comparisons have no meaning. Perhaps seeing these words spill out onto a printed page will be the catharsis I need. In that case thank you from my heart, for plowing through these pages with me as I put my life in order.

END

EPILOGUE

Genevieve is sixteen now, a time when teenagers are either heaven or hell, or perhaps a bit of both, and I am blessed with the former. We are having the happiest time in our lives since the short years of family life with her Dad came to an end.

My temper has melted away in the face of focusing on the wonderful things in our lives. Gen's occasional reversions to her old rude self don't get a rise out of me…in fact they make me smile, although I would never let her see. She is less Goldilocks - very very good, or very bad—and more Sunshine.

She is less moody, as am I, and we have both become more loving and relaxed. It has taken several months to reach this détente… such a short time compared to the years of angst we have overcome.

In the context of truthfulness that has been the theme of these pages, I am slightly reluctant, but not ashamed, to admit that I was aided immeasurably (I mean that in the true sense of the word, I have no idea how much or how little) by the use of Prozac for three months.

Just that short time was enough to give us the break we needed to regroup, to let my brain unwind, to see that I could indeed drop the hostile reactions, that this was truly a safe time and place to try a "no fear" stance. I have no idea how long it would have taken to come this far on my own, but seeing the results, I am thankful the drug was available.

Having always been leery of drugs of any kind (Aspirin is my idea of a great drug), I had adamantly resisted taking Prozac until the day my doctor in Marsh Harbour mentioned, "It's odd, I've noticed that people who could benefit from an antidepressant often will not take them, while others are happy to slurp them down like candy." That sounded like a challenge to me, one I accepted. We compromised, I said I would try it, but not for very long, and only every other day, not daily. This did not satisfy the doctor, but made sense to me.

Something produced a miracle. I do not know what percent was the Prozac, what percent was my decision to focus on enjoying my daughter rather than struggling with her, or the move from Nassau to this lovely place, or the joy of not having to work so hard to keep afloat financially, or the prayers… whatever the varying percentages, the whole came up to *100% magic.*

Seeing that all was going well on Prozac, it was an interesting decision to stop taking it…actually quite scary. What if I reverted to the impatient, easily provoked (yet unfailingly kind and funny!) person we had been living with before? I was relieved to find that the real me, no pills, was still me…but now without the quick temper, and a more laid back attitude…life is good.

* * * * *

It is Genevieve's high school graduation ceremony today, and we are at her school in Canada. Pomp, Circumstance, and Bagpipes. Her Dad has blessed us with his presence, and I mean that in the literal sense… I was so grateful he made the trip to St. Catherines for her special day, I could have kissed him. Gen's dimples beamed the entire day.

We sat together in the lovely stone Chapel for the parent student service. When the choir sent its glorious notes spiraling up to the arched beams and the stained glass windows, Gen shyly slipped her arm through mine, then through her Dad's on the other side, and just glowed.

It was the first time the three of us were together in over thirteen years, and it was so very important to her. I don't know if her Dad has any idea how much it meant to her that he was there, and to me to see our child so very happy. He was there for the handing out of the diplomas, he was there for the father-daughter dance. Finally, he was there for her.

My Gen girl now sixteen and graduated from high school. A commonplace milestone for many families perhaps, but for me a time to thank God, to laugh, to throw the proverbial hat in the air. I feel as if I have run a good race, done my best, and placed well near the front.

* * * * *

My very good friend David is staying with us for a few days in Hopetown, spending every daylight hour catching the surf thrown up by the last big storm. We have been friends for years, and his faults are twofold; he is too good looking to be true, and he is ten years younger than me. Soulful brown eyes, clever wit, tall, lean model's body, toned and buffed arms, and what my daughter would describe as a sixpack of rippling muscles for a stomach, he turns heads wherever he goes.

David strolled into my Nassau Restaurant alone one evening ten years ago after bringing a large yacht over from Fort Lauderdale to Hurricane hole Marina. It was my habit to visit every table for a chat to ascertain customers were happy, but before I had a chance to stop at this handsome stranger's table, he got up and started to walk out.

I intercepted him at the entrance, introduced myself as the owner, and asked why he was leaving. Too polite to give the real reason (was the waitress too slow, the music too loud? to this day I don't know) he simply said he'd, "changed his mind."

"No" I said, "That won't do, I will not have you walking out of my Restaurant without a good meal, my treat." I showed him to a preferred table, and assigned him a congenial waitress; a real "Bahama Mama" who danced and swayed to the music of our band as she dodged around the tables with trays loaded to the ceiling. This time I made it to his table for a chat over coffee, and we have been friends ever since.

I have asked him to read the first few pages of my writing, thinking to get a bit of constructive feedback that would be an indication whether to carry on, or bail out in the event the meanderings of my mind interest only me. I thought it would be quite easy to hand a few pages of my baby over to a friend, but it is a scary thrill waiting to see what he will say.

I find I can not read along with him in my mind, do not remember which thoughts are actually committed to paper and which are still in my head. Does he have the part about the fire? What about the Tibetan lamas, the lighthouse? Should I have asked him for constructive criticism only? No, I am glad I didn't put limits on his thinking, his response will be purely him, indicative of what one man thinks, giving me all manner of leeway to turn any negative response into something useful and positive.

Ten minutes, twenty minutes, a good sign, he is not skimming, he is *reading*. Finally the verdict, with a slightly surprised look… "I like it, it's good, I wish there was more to read now." Music to my ears, happy glow, great motivation to carry on.

The high is short lived, questions glimmer and flash in my mind. Would I have been felled by a lukewarm response? Or would I have been able, as I like to think, to pick myself up and use the criticism positively? Or would I have been crushed, and taken to my bed until a better bit of news came along, as my father did before me? More pressing, why do I want to know my reactions to a nonexistent negative response?

A sobering thought quiets the plethora of questions…I am not out of the woods yet, not by a long shot. The real test is yet to come. Friends are a safe barometer, I could maneuver around any grumbles on that front, but what will the weather be like with my pages in the hands of a stormy, impatient editor or publisher… a desk piled high with hopeful manuscripts?

Who am I to expect my pages to be dropped on the "OK" pile, followed by a short, lifechanging letter saying, "*We like it, we'll do it.*"

Yet as I write these words, I can see that happening. "*We like it, we'll do it.*" That is the thought I must keep. No fear; no What ifs, no why would I succeed where countless others have failed? Because with God's help I will make it happen.

I know God is here. He has made His presence felt to me in many small but important ways consistently since that very awesome proof many years ago, in the dining room of Chaban, when he let me know in no uncertain terms that someone cares for me. And when it happens, when these pages are being read by unknown eyes, and they like what they see… I will say once again "Thank You", and go on.

B. Benson

* * * * *

Note from the author, November 2010

Mark Twain's autobiography has just been released, 100 years after his death as he requested. He desired the freedom to write with the knowledge that anyone he put in his pages would not be alive at publication. He also would be "dead, and unaware, and indifferent..." and was therefore free to speak his "whole frank mind."

A noble thought, however one that by his documented struggles, did not make writing his memoirs any easier for him.

I am convulsed with laughter reading that while writing his autobiography over one hundred years ago Mark Twain grappled as I did with the dilemma of the compulsory 'Beginning, Middle and End' of a story... coming to the same conclusion I did...or vice versa.

After dozens of false starts and hundreds of pages, he determined that the 'Right Plan for telling the story of his life was to "Talk only about the thing which interests you for the moment, dropping it when its interest threatens to pale..." thus allowing his thoughts to 'range freely'. Mark Twain would "wander at free will all over his life, starting at no particular time."

Thank you Mark Twain for speaking clearly from the grave, giving 100 year old support to my theory that a memoir is a living thing that must be compelling and vivid, encompassing past reminiscences and current thoughts as they fly fresh from the brain... in whichever order they tumble... 'Beginning, Middle and End' be damned.

PHOTO GALLERY

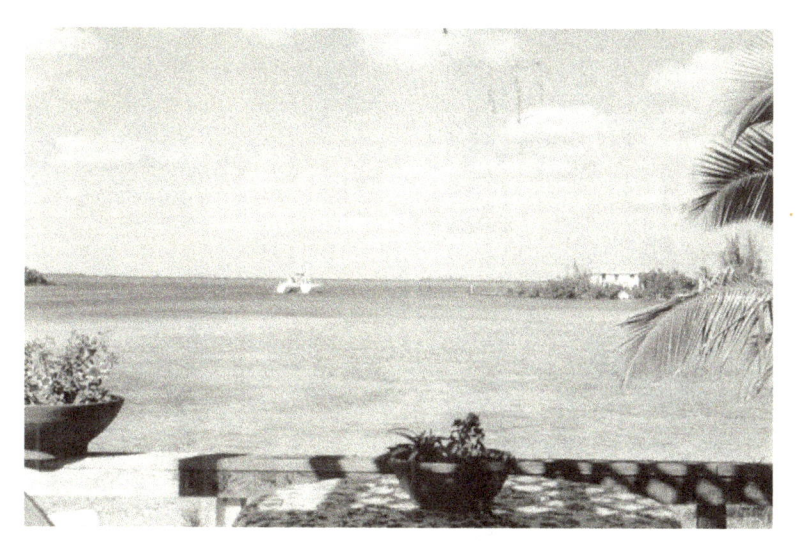

Lavender Cottage Deck, Harbor Entrance & Eagle Rock Island

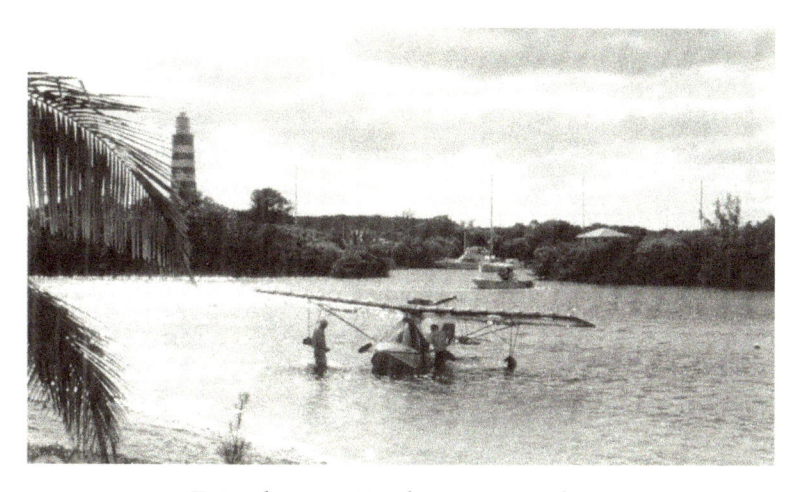

Friends stopping by…via seaplane

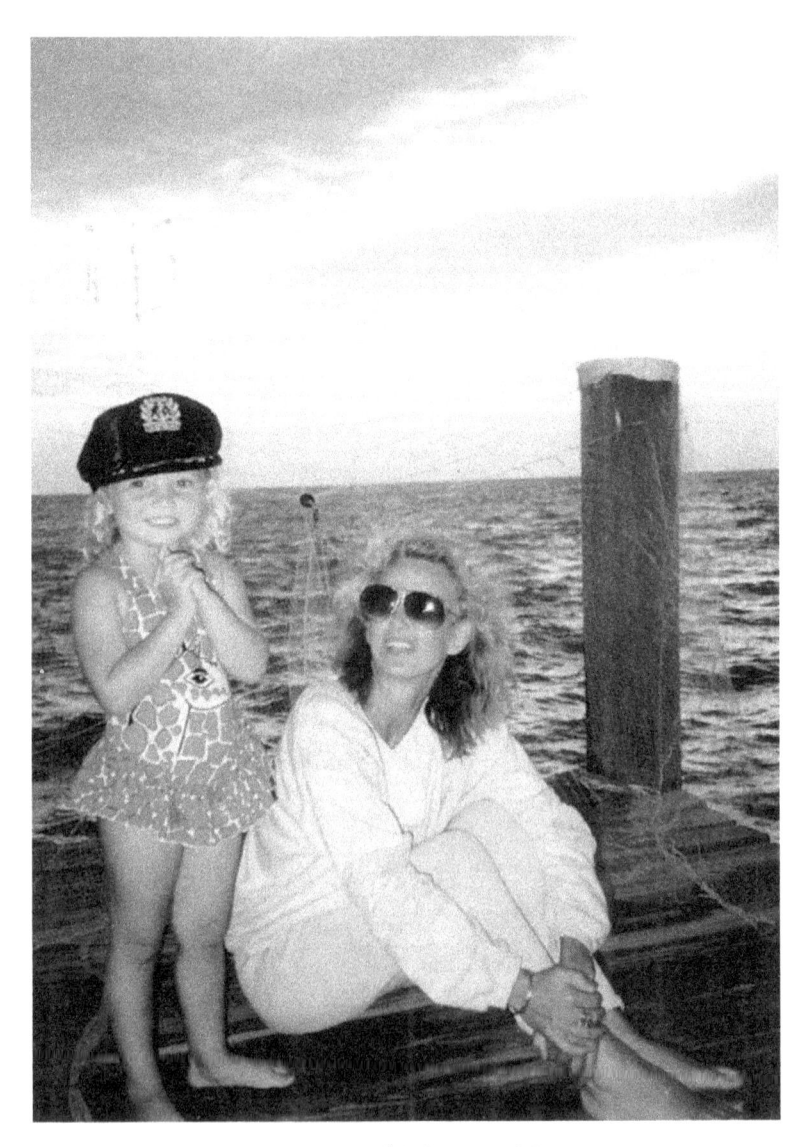

Genevieve and Mom in Nassau

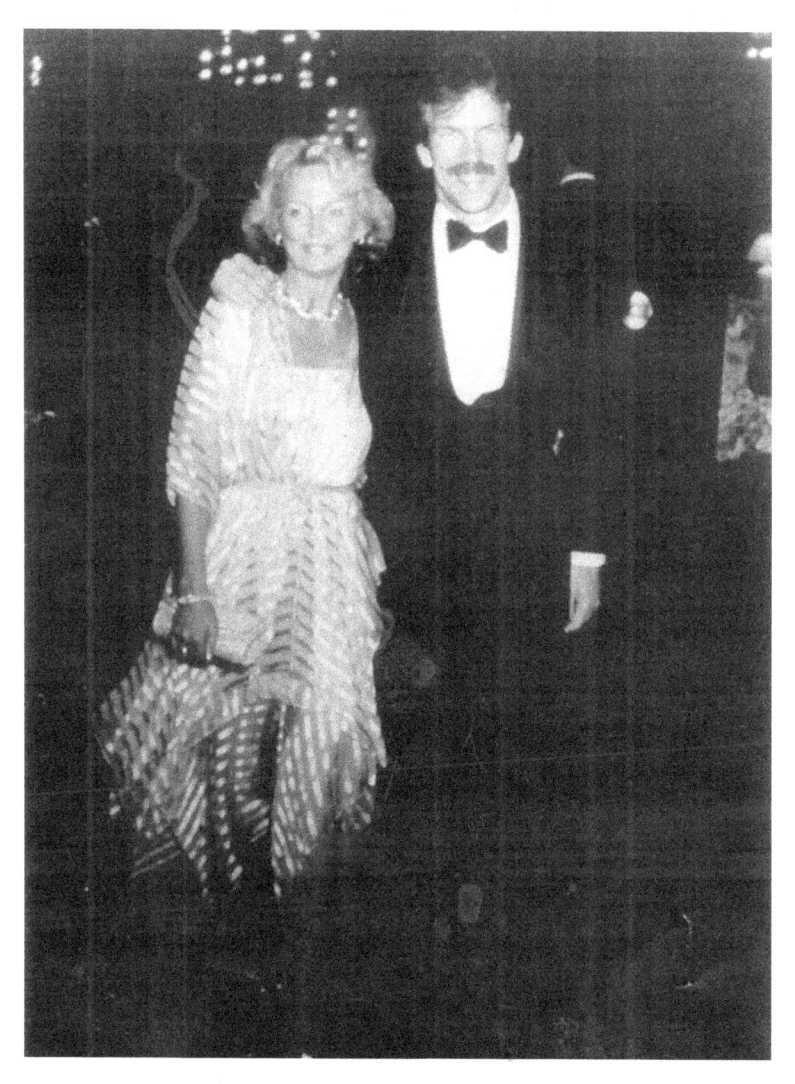

Gen's Mom and Dad in happier days

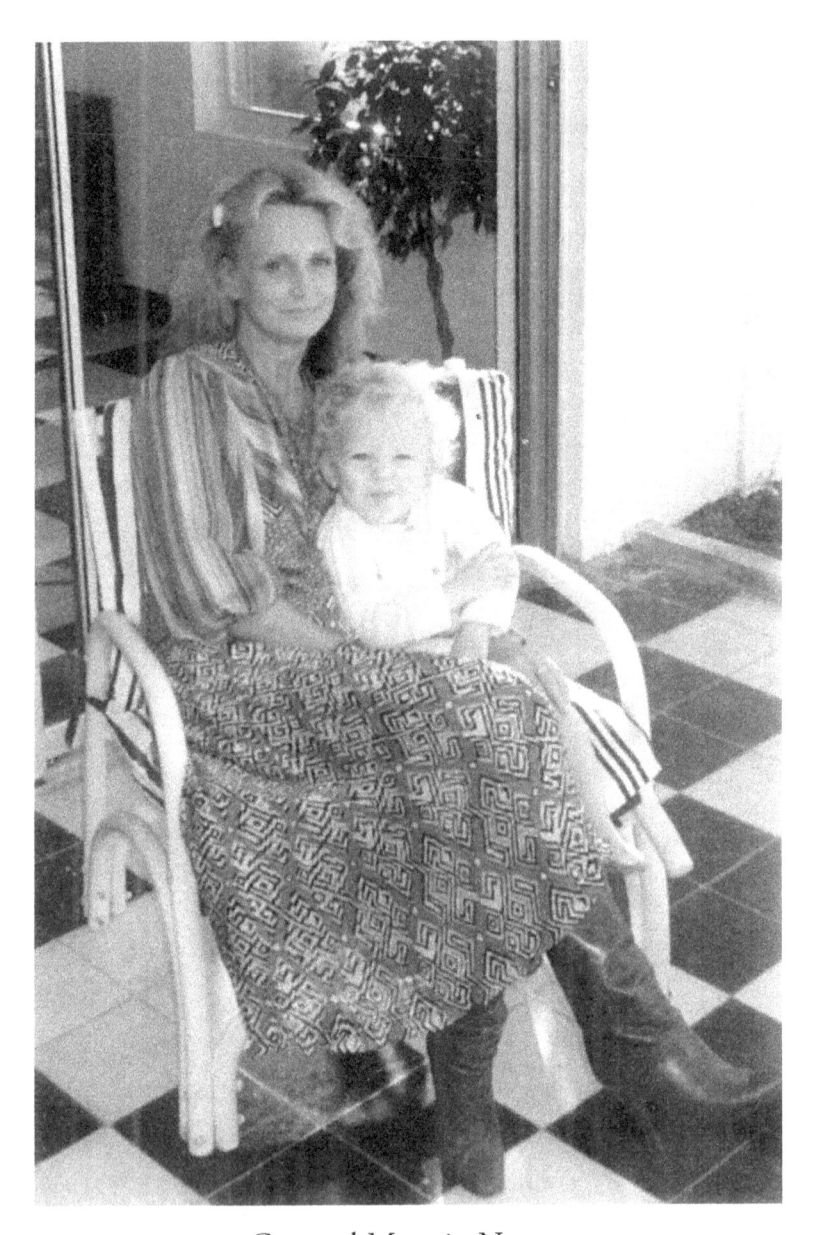

Gen and Mom in Nassau

Honey English

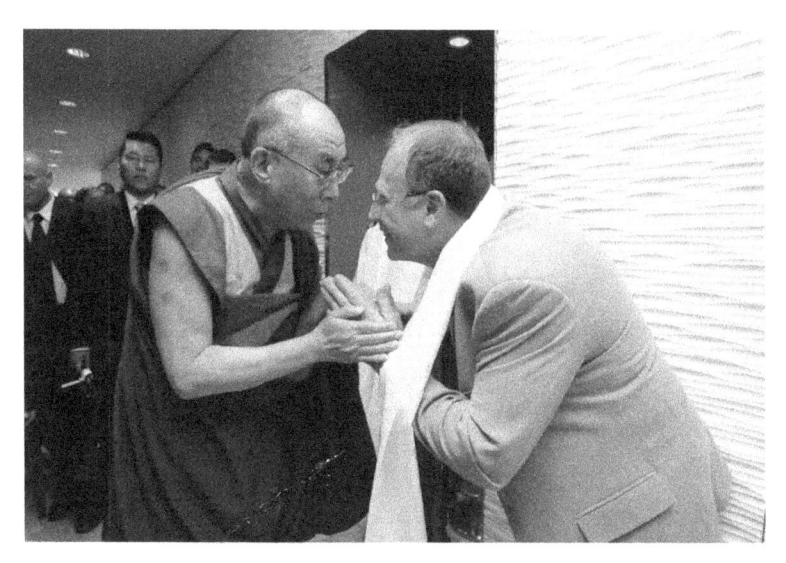

The Dalai Lama and my brother Kit

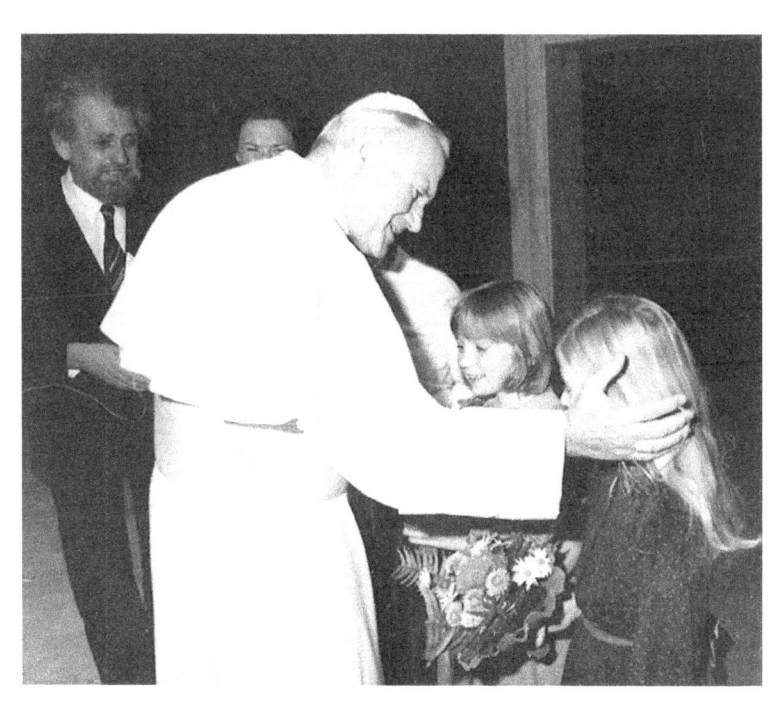

Private audience. Pope John Paul II, Father and two younger sisters

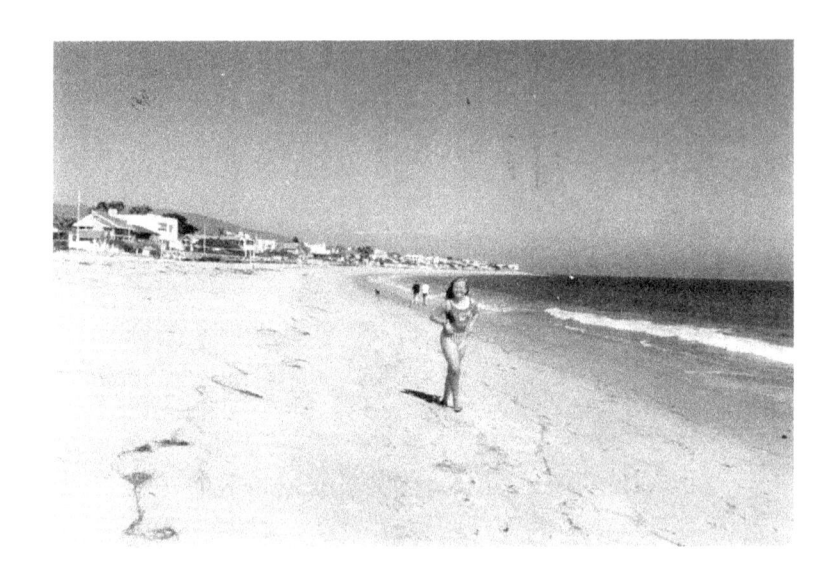

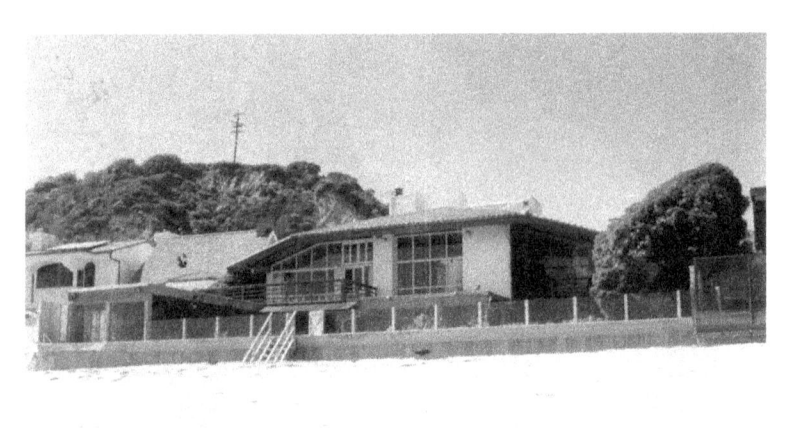

Gen, Malibu Colony Beach, and the 'Big House'

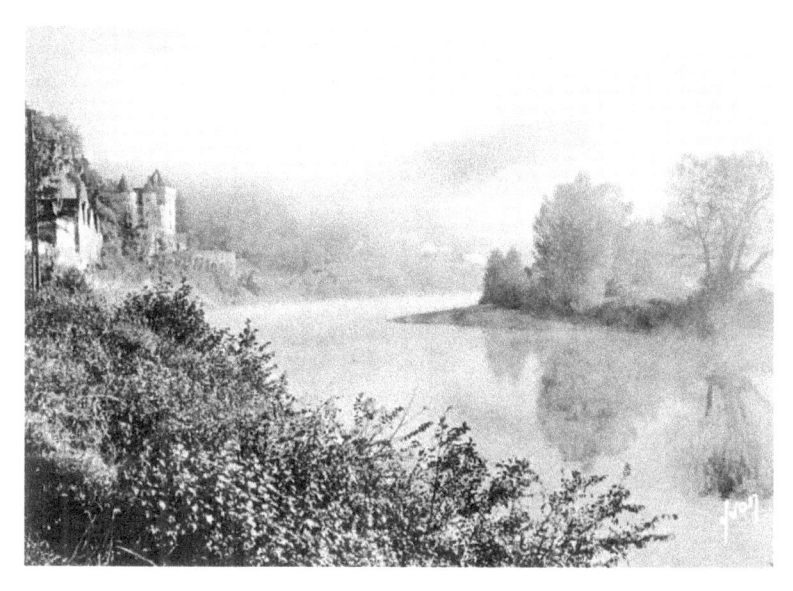

The Dordogne River under early morning mist

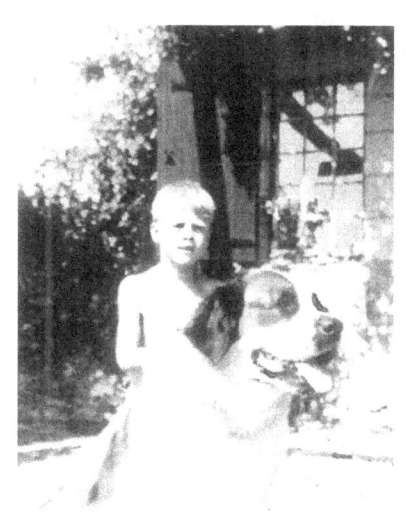

Little brother and 'Nana', the St. Bernard

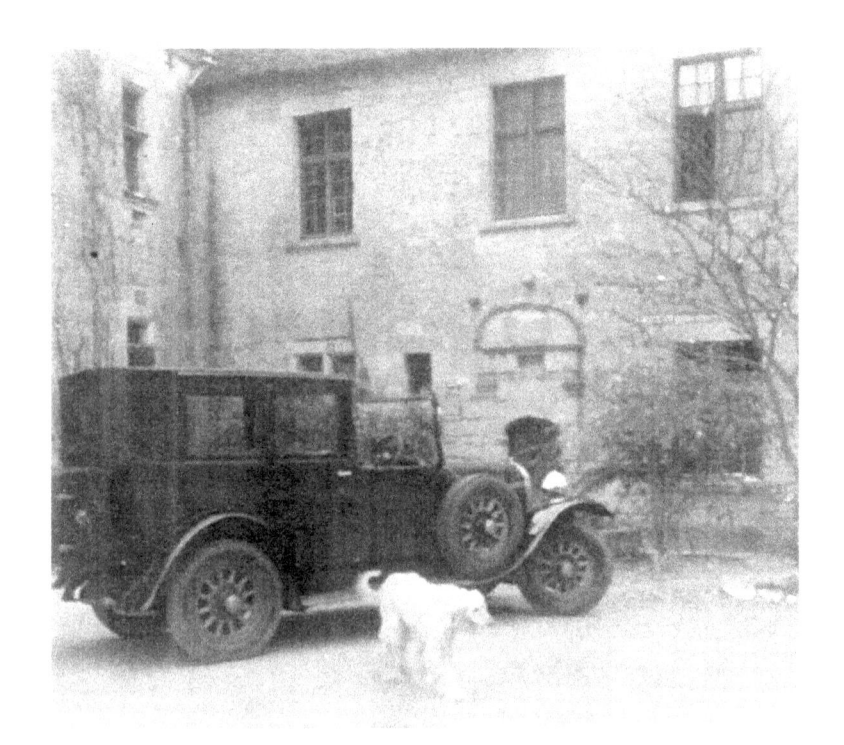

The Napier and an Afghan hound

Honey English

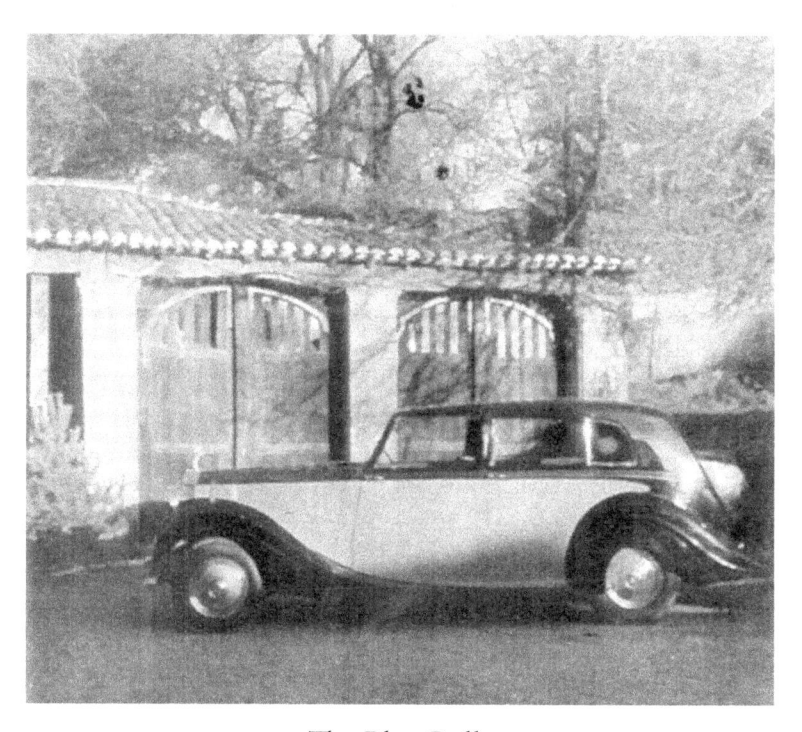

The Blue Rolls

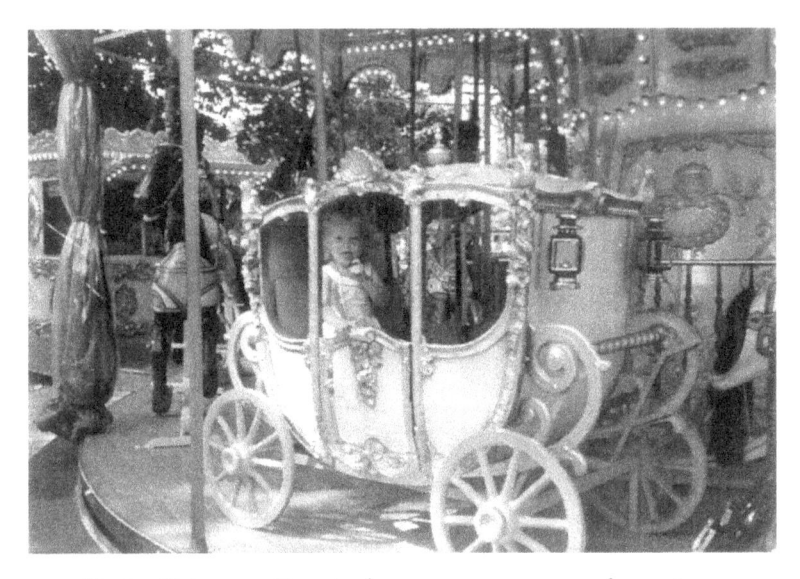

Paris, Princess Gen in her merry-go-round carriage

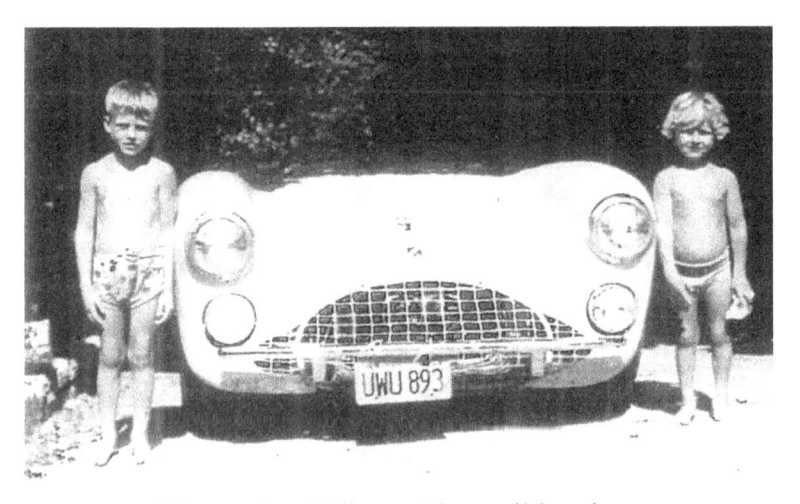

Blue racing Talbot with small brothers

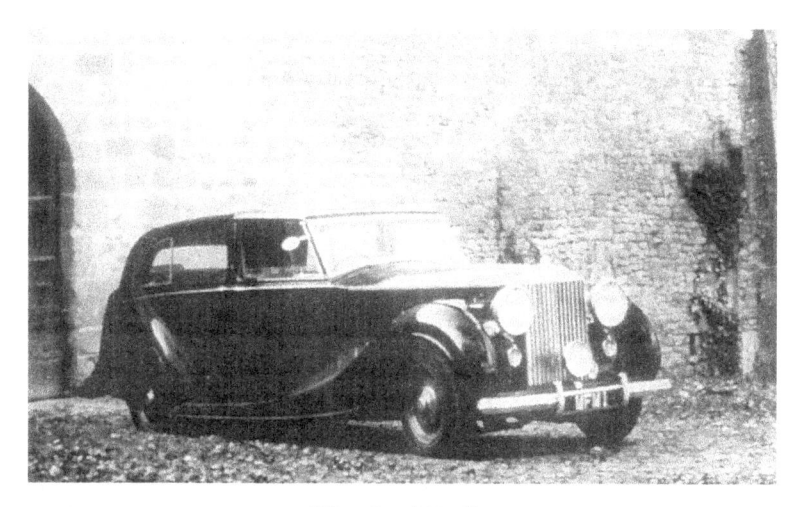

The Red Rolls

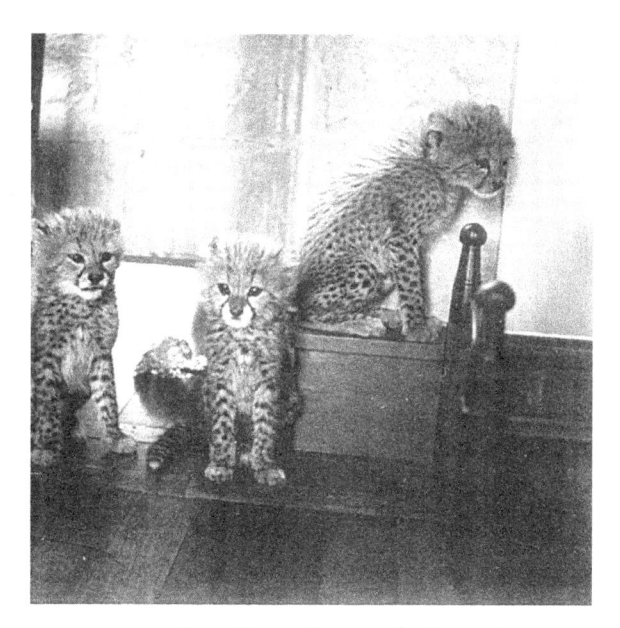

Baby Cheetahs at Chaban

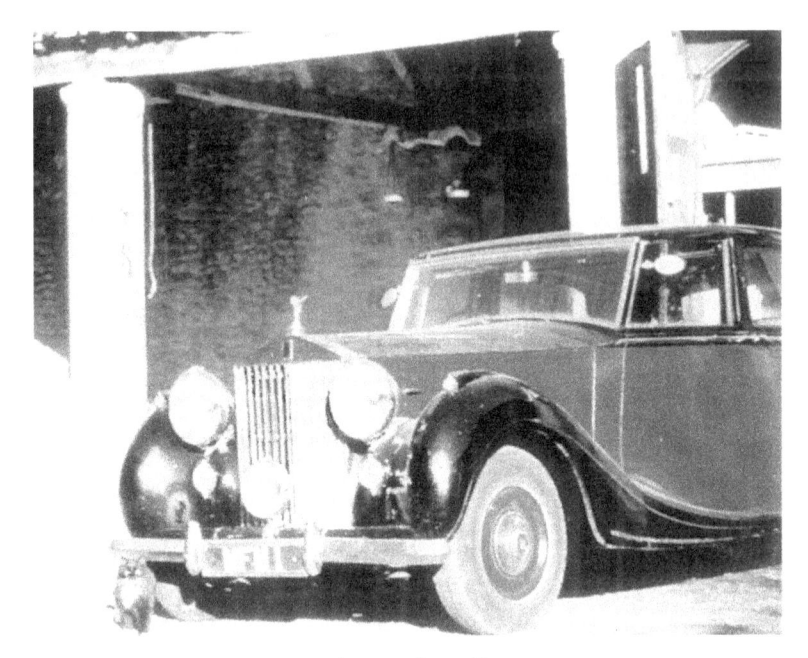

The Red Rolls

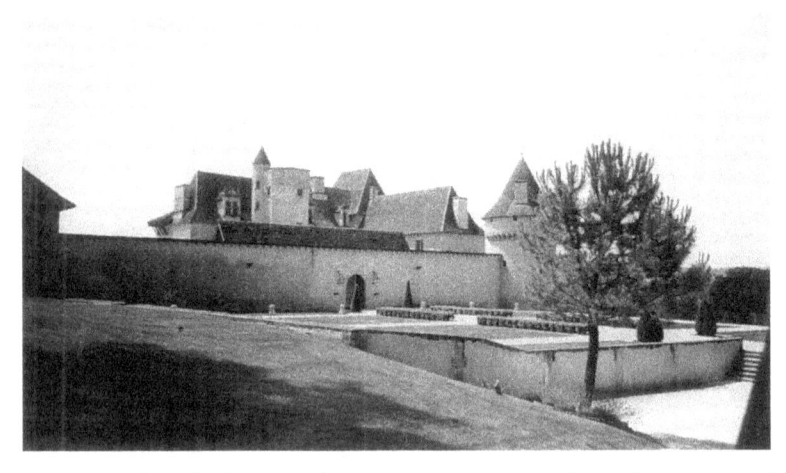

Chateau de Chaban, 13th Century tower and gardens retored
1996

Honey English

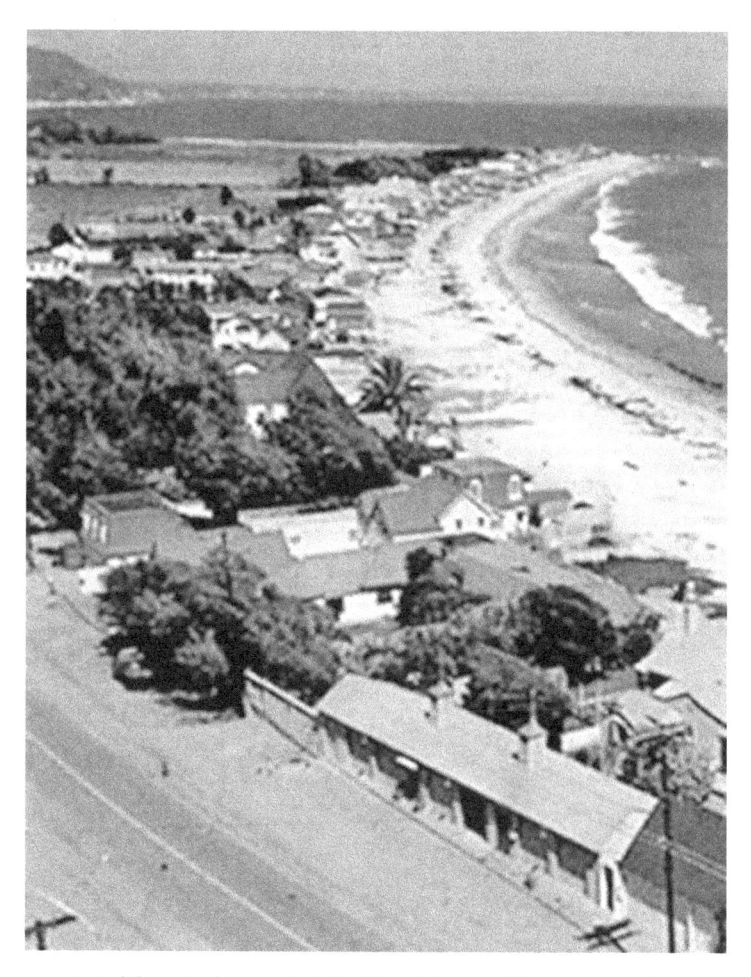

Malibu Colony 1960's 'Big House' bottom right

"It is my fervent wish that everyone in the world would open their hearts to let in the Little Boy of *The Peace Book*."
—His Holiness Pope John Paul II

"...(THE) PEACE BOOK expounds a significant message, highly cherished by all humanity... No doubt the concept of this great book will help contribute to peace in a way that touches the hearts of millions thirsty for seeing it established and widespread."
—Anwar el Sadat

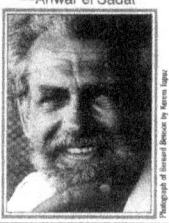

TO ALL OF THE CHILDREN OF THE WORLD, THIS BOOK IS DEDICATED. AND TO ALL OF THE BIG PEOPLE TOO.

"With simplicity and clarity, *The Peace Book* brings light and hope to a world filled with fear and despair. A little boy cries, 'I want to live!' and his innocence teaches us that peace is possible. This book is for all ages. Reading it will touch your heart and it could change (even *save*) your life by awakening love in a world that seems headed toward destruction."
—Gerald G. Jampolsky, M.D., author of the bestselling book *Love Is Letting Go Of Fear*

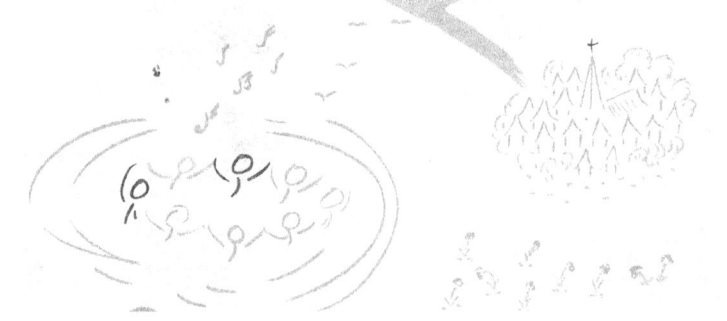

Back Cover of *The Peace Book* by Bernard Benson

FURTHER INFORMATION ON PEACE CHILD INTERNATIONAL

Peace Child International **http://www.peacechild.org/**

Beginnings - The Founders: 1981	
	Bernard Benson: Author, entrepreneur, artist, visionary, Bernard provided the story that became Peace Child. The idea of setting the story in the future and looking back to the past came from his landmark book, The Peace Book.
	David Gordon: Composer and lyricist, David's songs have been the lifeblood of Peace Child. David's oratorio Alpha Omega was an inspiration for the Peace Child musical. David is Cat Steven's brother.
	Michael and Eirwen Harbottle: Michael was an army Brigadier who became a UN Peace-keeping expert. Working with his wife Eirwen on the World Disarmament Campaign, they had the idea to put the Peace Book and Alpha Omega together and produce a "Celebration for Peace".

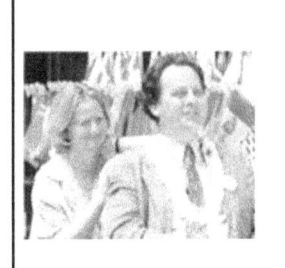

	David Woollcombe and Rosey Simonds: David wrote and directed the UK and USA Peace Child premieres at the Royal Albert Hall and Kennedy Centre which Rosey co-produced. Together they have run Peace Child International for the past 28 years.

Peace Child International is a Buntingford, UK based charity (UK Charity Registration number: 1095189) focusing on sustainable development and youth empowerment. http://www.peacechild.org/

History of the Organisation
From Wikipedia, the free encyclopedia

Peace Child International began as a musical**, based** on **Bernard Benson's *The Peace Book.*** The Musical itself was composed by David Gordon and written by David Woollcombe. It intended to resolve conflict between the USA and the USSR. Since its original use the musical has been used in conflict resolution efforts in Azerbaijan/Armenia, Central America, Cyprus, the former Yugoslavia, India, Israel and Northern Ireland Since 1992 Peace Child has focused mainly on the issue of sustainable development producing a number of books on the subject with UN agencies.

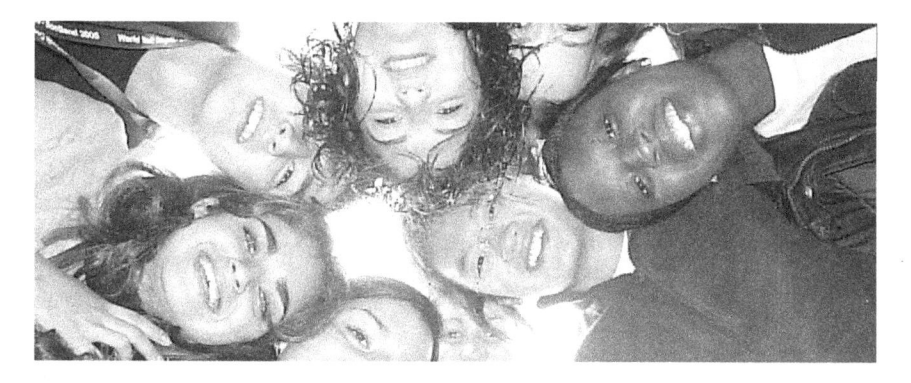

Peace Child International is registered in the UK as an educational charity, and since its founding in 1981 has grown to unite more than 1,500 affiliate groups and networks in over 180 countries.

Peace Child's mission is to **empower young people to be the change they want to see in the world**. This theme is at the forefront of each of our projects and programs, and is the standard by which we work. PCI supports young people around the world to produce books, musicals, educational materials, workshops and training courses on their major generational challenges: climate change, peace, human rights, poverty, and sustainable development. PCI also funds young people to undertake community-based action projects of their own through the "Be the Change!" program, and hosts the bi-annual World and European Youth Congress series.

ABOUT THE AUTHOR:

Writing stories since childhood to record the fanciful adventures of her avant-garde family members, Bernadette inherited a strong literary background from her grandfather, **Robert Saville-Sneath**, author of the earliest book on Airplane Recogniton during World War II, special Penguin edition. Her father, **Bernard Benson**, wrote and illustrated *The Peace Book* in 1981.

His Holiness Pope John Paul II gave Bernard a private audience after reading *The Peace Book*, and is quoted on the back cover; "It is my fervent wish that everyone in the world would open their hearts to let in the Little Boy of *The Peace Book*"

Anwar el Sadat also gives a testimonial, as well as **Gerald G. Jampolsky**, M.D., author of **Letting Go of Fear.**

Bernadette attended the musical performance of *The Peace Book* with her father at London's Royal Albert Hall in 1982, entitled The Peace Child. Susannah York was the Storyteller, the music was written by Cat Steven's brother David Gordon, and a talented group of children was chosen to perform the musical. The production was a sellout success, and a second musical was held at Washington DC's Kennedy Center.

The Peace Book has become a much loved classic, and was the motivating force behind the foundation of Peace Child International. Twenty eight years later this non-profit organization continues to, *'Empower young people to BE the change they want to SEE in the world'*

…through musicals, theatre, and education and collaboration with the UN. Both the book and the musicals are credited with being part of the effort to bring about the end of the Cold War with Russia. Bernadette was born in England, raised in California and France. She spent fifteen years in the Bahamas with her daughter Genevieve and now resides in Westport, Massachusetts.

To Contact Author: BIBI@Girlstocks.com

CPSIA information can be obtained
at www.ICGtesting.com
Printed in the USA
BVHW040737070522
636391BV00001B/11

9 781456 769499